Sex Education
Is for the Family

Other Zondervan Books by Tim LaHaye . . .

SEX
EDUCATION
IS FOR THE FAMILY

Tim LaHaye

PYRANEE BOOKS
ZONDERVAN PUBLISHING HOUSE
GRAND RAPIDS, MICHIGAN

Sex Education Is for the Family

Pyranee Books are published by the Zondervan Publishing House
1415 Lake Drive, S.E., Grand Rapids, Michigan 49506

Library of Congress Cataloging in Publication Data

LaHaye, Tim F.
    Sex education is for the family.

    "Pyranee books."
    1. Sex—Religious aspects—Christianity. 2. Family—Religious life.
I. Title.
BT708.L425   1985   241'.66   85-14379
ISBN 0-310-27010-3

All Scripture quotations, unless otherwise noted, are taken from the HOLY
BIBLE: NEW INTERNATIONAL VERSION (North American Edition). Copy-
right © 1978 by the International Bible Society. Used by permission of
Zondervan Bible Publishers.

Printed in the United States of America

85 86 87 88 89 90 / 10 9 8 7 6 5 4 3 2 1

Dedicated to all parents who want to teach their own children about sex but are hesitant to proceed. It is hoped that this book will remove your fear and arm you with sufficient knowledge so that you can impart crucial information concerning this most important subject with confidence. Remember, a clear understanding of his sexuality will affect almost everything else in your child's life.

Contents

In Appreciation

The author acknowledges the help of many researchers and other writers in the preparation of this manuscript. Particular appreciation is extended to Frank York, Sherry Barnes, and my artist, Carol Tubbs.

Introduction

SEX, SEXUALITY, morality, conception, abortion, homosexuality—these are highly sensitized words that need to be defined even for young children. But whose job is that? Does it belong to the school, the government, or the church? Independent agencies like Planned Parenthood? The family?

I believe that God has given the responsibility for sex education to the family. Without parental permission, any other instruction on these subjects is a gross invasion of family rights and privacy.

Yet our public schools insist that they teach sex education "because the parents fail to do so" or "because the parents want us to." Others say, "We teach sex ed in an attempt to halt the growing problem of teenage pregnancy and venereal disease."

As a concerned student of sex education, which has been taught in our government-controlled schools for more than twenty years, I do not hesitate to declare all of these assertions untrue. In fact, the explicit form of radical sex education now practiced by our government schools usurps the rights of the family and has directly contributed to the increase in both teenage promiscuity and unwed pregnancy.

Why should you as a parent teach your children about sex? Because it is probably the most important subject in their lives, primarily because their attitudes toward sex will affect almost every other part of their being. It is imperative that they develop the right attitude toward this subject, and you are the most influential people in their world. They will accept the truth about sex from parents more readily than from anyone else. Moreover, sexual information is best shared with little children as their interest grows, and we are the only people who spend sufficient quality time with them to provide just enough information to satisfy their curiosity on a given point when they need it.

Formal classes on human sexuality tend to create an abnormal obsession with sex in the mind of children when they should be curious about many other things in life. Such classes dump too much information on children long before they need it and often at a time when they are not interested. A number of critics have warned that it can be dangerous to arouse a concern for this subject when there is no natural interest.

Parents who talk to their own children about sex create a natural context for it that helps to prevent unhealthy curiosity. In addition, it provides for us as parents—the God-appointed people in our children's lives—the opportunity to teach them our moral values. It is extremely dangerous when the sex educator at school reflects a value system that conflicts with that of the parents.

Our values and a healthy outlook on sexuality will enable our children to reach adulthood with a sound basis for making major decisions relative to dating, courtship, and marriage. In the process of growing up, they will develop a healthy attitude toward the sexuality of their brothers, sisters, and friends. Our instruction will enable them spiritually to establish a proper place for sex in their lives so that they can minimize those thoughts and activities that produce guilt. Unless guilt feelings are dealt with properly, they will hinder a child's spiritual development.

Unfortunately, most parents are afraid to teach their own children about sex. Somehow we have been brainwashed into thinking that parents "aren't qualified" to address this delicate subject. That is nonsense. Most parents know more about sex education than they realize, even if they are rusty on the proper names for the various parts and functions of the body. This book is designed to give courage and insight to parents by teaching them what their children need to know at the time they need to know it so that they can become the primary sex education teachers of their children.

1

Who Should Teach Sex Education?

WE MAY BE AS certain as death and taxes that someone is going to teach our children about sex. It could be the dirty little kid down the street who knows everything that is wrong and ugly. It may be the cable TV program that's turned on some night when we're not home. Or possibly a secular humanist evangelist of sex education in the public school who does not share our moral values and will serve as a self-appointed guru of sexuality. It may even be a child molester. If we as parents do not teach our children about sex, they will probably gain information from the wrong source.

Sex is the most difficult subject in the world to discuss, and most people either avoid it or inject humor into the conversation, lowering the discussion to an unsavory level or reducing its significance. In most cases, parents—even good parents who responsibly teach their children about everything else they should know—somehow tend to avoid the issue of sex altogether.

Sex is such an intimate subject that it usually produces a strong emotional reaction, depending on a person's background. If you were not introduced to it casually and respectfully by your parents, you will probably find it difficult to discuss objectively. But you can learn to treat it like other significant matters and incorporate it into the training of your children. If it is "embarrassing" or "difficult" and you ignore it as so many parents do, your decision may be fatal to your children—or it may cause them to enter marriage already pregnant or emotionally and mentally crippled.

In the history of the world, it has never been more imperative that children gain information about sex at an early age. No matter how much we try, we cannot prevent even young children from learning about the subject long before they need to. Thus the sex education of children by their parents becomes a matter of self-defense. We can only be sure our children learn the essential facts together with moral values if we serve as the instructors ourselves. We must not leave this vital task to others, for in so doing we risk leaving our children vulnerable to sexual exploitation. In fact, we should assume in this sex-crazed day that our children will eventually be confronted with sexual temptation. The only safeguard is parental preparation for that day. Most exploitation of children could be avoided by mental and moral training.

Parents may fail to teach their children about sex because they do not feel qualified. One mother asked, "Who am *I* to teach my child about sex?" I answered, "Her parent!" That is our primary qualification. This sincere mother clearly wanted the best for her daughter, but she made a common mistake. She thought that comprehensive knowledge about sexuality was the major requirement for being her child's educator. She did not understand that a little research, as in reading this book, could make up for her deficiencies while still safeguarding the central point of sex education—teaching moral values.

One of the time-honored rights of parents in this country is teaching moral values to their children. Some in education and government, however, consider it *their* right; thus they are doing everything in their power to impose amorality on children. Surrender of our parental rights will guarantee the loss of our children, who are our most important possession. This book is dedicated to putting the essentials of sex into the hands of parents so they can teach their sons and daughters the facts they need *and* the moral values that must accompany this information.

CAN WE TRUST THE PUBLIC SCHOOLS TO TEACH OUR CHILDREN ABOUT SEX?

There was a day, more than twenty years ago, when the public schools taught personal hygiene as part of the physical education program. These gender-segregated classes spent more time on morality and chastity than sexuality. I well remember my sex education in the eighth grade. As we dressed for gym class, our "coach," a Roman Catholic father of seven, overheard one of the boys say something dirty. He angrily lined us up and proceeded to pace up and down the floor while lecturing us about "the facts of life." I recall how that good man, whom I admired, stressed respect for girls and womanhood, self-control, mental purity, and other important attitudes that stood me in good stead throughout my days in the army and prepared me for marriage.

Unfortunately, that kind of teaching in the public schools is rare today. Thanks to the U.S. Supreme Court's exclusion of prayer, the Bible, religion, and moral values from our schools and thanks to the institutionalizing of sex education by secular humanist educators, we have now created an obsession with sex among far too many of our nation's forty-three million public-school children.

Schools, of course, are not all alike. Occasionally I hear of a courageous school superintendent or principal who understands the harmful effects of secular humanism on the learning process and consciously fights against it. One admitted recently, however, "It is getting harder all the time." The SIECUS (Sex Information and Educational Council of the United States) brand of sex education has swept the country, bringing explicit sex instruction into many classrooms and inundating our children with information they are ill-prepared to digest.

It is interesting to note that during the same period when radical sex education material has infiltrated most schools from kindergarten through the twelfth grade, there has been a drastic decline in learning. It is a well-publicized fact that SAT (Standard Achievement Test) scores reveal that today's children may know more about sex than reading, writing, spelling and math.*

THE CASE AGAINST SEX EDUCATION IN PUBLIC SCHOOLS

For more than 175 years, American public schools included few or no formal sex education classes. If the subject was taught at all, it appeared in conjunction with physical education or biology. Now, however, many schools offer two-or-three-week sessions every year for twelve years. Having lectured hundreds of times on the subject and having written a best-selling book on sexual adjustment in marriage, I believe we can teach most people all the basic ingredients in two or three hours just prior to marriage.** One hour of instruction a day, five days a week, for three weeks a year times twelve years equals 180 hours. That is not education; it amounts to indoctrination of young people that easily leads to an obsession. But the amount of time devoted to this in the classroom is not my only objection to sex education in public schools.

---

*For a thorough treatment of this subject, read the author's book, *The Battle for the Public Schools* (Old Tappan, N.J.: Fleming H. Revell, 1983), which documents the explicit sex education teaching in our schools and its harmful effects on children's morals and learning ability.

**See *The Act of Marriage* (Grand Rapids: Zondervan, 1976), co-authored by Tim and Beverly LaHaye.

1. Public Schools Teach Sex
Without Moral Values

The secular humanists who control SIECUS and Planned Parenthood (organizations that frequently provide lecturers for schools) and a large percentage of the curriculum designers are evolutionists. Many are also atheists. Why is that important? Because an atheistic evolutionist considers man an animal that does not possess an innate conscience and is not responsible to God for his behavior. He rejects moral absolutes, insisting that each generation establish its own judgments of right and wrong. In fact, modern education repeatedly affirms that "there are no rights and wrongs." Nowhere is that false notion more harmful than in the sex-education classroom.

Moral absolutes do exist. The Bible clearly validates rights and wrongs, and 75-to-85 percent of Americans accept biblical standards as the model for behavior. Yet many of our tax-supported public-school sex-education teachers regard our children as animals who should "practice their sexuality" or "do their own thing." They seem obsessed with the idea that it is their responsibility to teach our young "all the facts" and let them make up their own minds about right and wrong—whether parents like it or not.

Teaching sex education in mixed classes to hot-blooded teenagers without benefit of moral values is like pouring gasoline on emotional fires. An explosion is inevitable.

The enjoyment of sexual relations is and, for morally minded people, always has been an adult experience. Furthermore, our culture has consistently taught that individuals should not engage in intercourse until the participants are willing to take responsibility for their actions—in other words, become parents. Sexual activity will eventually lead to parenthood, as any of the more than one million pregnant, unwed schools girls in America each year will testify. Who authorized these self-styled "sexologists" to teach our children otherwise? Who elected them to change our centuries-old tradition that left sexual matters in the domain of the family? Who commissioned them to usurp the role of parents? Admittedly, not all sex educators openly advocate that teenagers become promiscuous, but few teach the biblical injunction "Flee youthful lusts."

When the U.S. Supreme Court outlawed prayer and the Bible, the secular humanists in education seized the occasion to change traditional practices of teaching a value-laden education. They have told me, "Since religion has been expelled from our schools, so have God and morality." In other words, since morals are based on religion and since religion is no longer acceptable in our government-controlled schools, neither are moral values. Therefore, moral values may no longer be taught in many of our nation's schools.

Offering explicit sex education *without* moral values is worse than not teaching it at all, for it leads to experimentation with little or no restraint.

2. Sex Education Is Too Explicit

I led a campaign in California several years ago that helped to halt a radical course on sex education for kindergarten through grade twelve that was unbelievably explicit. Financed by the federal government to the tune of $175,000, the program shocked everyone with standards of decency. Believe it or not, it called for the teaching of the details of intercourse to kindergartners. I have yet to meet a parent who wasn't incensed upon seeing the explicit nature of the material. (The current policy in many schools is to keep parents uninformed about what goes on behind the classroom doors.)

That single course, designed by "sexologists" employed at taxpayers' expense and taught to the state's sex-education instructors, proves one thing: We cannot trust the schools to formulate a sane and responsible form of sex education without close scrutiny by parents. In essence, we cannot rely on our educators to protect the innocent minds of our children. Not all public educators are corrupt, of course, but the public has ample reason to distrust many of those in charge of such programs.

In my opinion, when some humanist sex educators refer to "teaching sex education," they really mean instructing young people in "the art of intercourse." Parents almost never mean that. In September 1979 a report entitled "The Impact of Life Science Instruction at George Mason High School, Falls Church, Virginia" was released by Columbia University. Financed by a grant from the Ford-Rockefeller Program in Population Policy, it exposed the *real* goal of most humanist sex educators. Summing up the in-depth study, the report said, ". . . One goal of the sex education program is to alert students to the probabilities of pregnancy *and encourage only responsible sexual intercourse,* using contraception, if such sexual activity occurs at all" (author's italics).

Parents usually understand the term "sex education" to mean that their children need to know about hygiene, their own sexuality, and the fact that sex is to be reserved for marriage. The outcries of parental groups enraged by the advanced subject material taught to their children clearly indicate that some instructors use the public-school sex-education classroom to teach intercourse long before young people are old enough to bear the responsibilities for their actions. Recent surveys of today's high school students show that they are much more sexually active than when the current sex-education courses were introduced.

Until public educators recognize that teaching intercourse without benefit of moral values is overstepping their authority, parents should prepare themselves to offer proper information within the sanctity of the home.

3. Sex Education in Mixed Classes Should Be Forbidden

If explicit sexual information must be taught in public-school classrooms, it certainly should not be presented in mixed classes. A certain feminine mystique or modesty is broken down when thirty high schoolers including both boys and girls study this subject together. Sex is and always should be an intensely private subject. Teaching it in mixed classes makes it cruelly public and reduces it to a common level.

In addition, such classes are vulnerable to the class jester with perverted morals. A dirty comment here or an off-color response there further serves to break down the natural reserve between the sexes. Public schools are noted for "rap" sessions, or question periods after lectures. The question-and-answer sessions that I have conducted suggest that not all questions that come into a person's mind are appropriate for public discussion.

Female periods, ovulation, abortion, birth control, wet dreams, testicles, or ejaculation may be appropriate subjects for high school juniors and seniors, but certainly not in mixed classes. I do not conceive any moral good that can come from discussions on these subjects in mixed classes, but I can anticipate much harm from them. Sex education that lowers the privacy level of sex can do more harm than good, for it reduces the sex act to the level of animal instinct—which is where a humanistic sexologist perceives it.

4. Sex Education Classes Show Little Regard for Individual Differences

Children do not mature at the same rate, and that is a major problem in public education. Some ninth-graders act like elementary students, while others try to impersonate college freshmen. Consequently, some may be ready to consider aspects on human sexuality at their grade level, while others are not.

A doctor friend of mine has a daughter who began to develop physically when she was thirteen years old. When his wife suggested that they should go shopping for a bra, the sensitive girl became so upset that she ran into the bathroom and cried. Can you imagine such a girl being humiliated in a mixed class on sex education with its raucous laughter? For some reason, public-school administrators want to institute elaborate systems and curricula respecting student individuality—except on the subject of sex.

5. Sex Education Can Create an Obsession With Sex Among Youth

A typical junior high or high school student does not need his interest in sex artificially stimulated. New forces within his body are making him sexually conscious and responsive. In addition, television, magazines, and other influences in society serve as major sources of sexual stimulation. An adolescent doesn't need the added stimulus of sex instruction in mixed classes.

Dr. James Parsons, a Christian psychologist in Florida who has debated the Who's Who in Modern Sexology, has come to the conclusion that "Modern sex education is creating such an obsession with sex that it leaves the student little time or interest in either spiritual or academic pursuits." Who is to say that some secular-humanist sex educators don't have that intent? High school young people need only one obsession to prepare them for life: an obsession with learning about God, man, the universe, and the skills necessary to prepare them to reach their God-given potential.

6. Sex Education Should Contain Instruction on Self-Control and Responsibility, Not Self-Indulgence or Pleasure

God gave us the gift of sexuality as a means of blessing to married couples. Its two primary purposes are propagation of the race and mutual pleasure. It cannot legitimately be taught to unwed teenagers for either purpose. Yet public schools insist upon their right "to teach it all" (usually prematurely) without including aspects such as responsibility and self-control.

A fifteen-year-old-boy may be physically old enough to impregnate a girl, but he is hardly old enough to provide for a child. Who has ever accused the public schools of teaching such a youth that the results of sex are his responsibility? No, the approach seems to establish sex without responsibility—or recourse to contraceptives, abortion, or public welfare support. Teaching on self-control and responsibility would have a chilling effect on youthful passions. I have never heard of anyone being psychologically, physically, or socially damaged by the application of self-control in the face of sexual temptation. That would, of course, require programming the mind in advance with moral values.

Public schools seem to pose a peculiar problem with moral values. Although many individual teachers reflect a strong commitment to moral values personally, most "educrats" (the national leaders of education) disallow them a place for such teachings in public schools. They usually equate moral values with religion and expel them; consequently, teachers are able to teach "situation ethics" or their own values in the name of "academic freedom." Little or no concern is given to parental values, particularly the value that their children remain virginal until marriage. The God-given right to instill values in their own children is one more reason why sex education should be taught by parents. Perhaps that is why increasing numbers of Christian parents are sending their children to Christian schools or providing sex education at home.

7. A Moral Holocaust Has Resulted From the Past Twenty Years of Sex Education

Twenty years ago I warned the local school board that introducing the new SIECUS program of sex education would create a wave of promiscuity, teenage pregnancies, and venereal disease. I was ridiculed. Today that list comprises the most serious problems on the high school level. Genital herpes, a venereal disease that has already claimed more than twenty-one million victims, has created a moral backlash. After two decades during which more than 60 percent of high school students became promiscuous, there is a new interest in moral purity on the part of many young people. It is hoped this will offset the artificially stimulating sexual instruction that infests too many schools.

Sex education in the schools was promoted to parents as a means of solving social problems. However, the obsession with sex created by such classes has more than doubled the problems they promised to solve—which is typical of godless humanism's solutions to anything. It solves nothing but instead compounds the dilemma.

Children are born with two parents who are responsible to teach them about sex. The parents should never delegate that responsibility to a stranger, particularly one who teaches in an environment that is hostile to religion and moral values.

Few aspects of a person's life have greater impact on his future happiness than his sexuality. If he starts out improperly and becomes promiscuous, it will take divine forgiveness and several years to undo the consequences. In some cases, the results are irreversible.

Parents need to guard their children's sexuality and all teachings on that subject. No one has a greater stake in the future happiness, success, and development of a child than his parents. That is why parents should be the sex educators of their own children.

Unfortunately, most parents don't know how to teach their children about sex, and that is the reason for this book. Any parent willing to use this book as a manual, appropriate to the age of his child, can be armed with what he needs to teach his own child. Sex education is really for the family. This book will help you keep it that way and still ensure that your child gains all the necessary information he needs for his age from a Christian perspective.

2

Babies—Innocent, But Curious

SEX EDUCATION begins before birth. Scientists are now discovering that unborn babies are aware of their surroundings and can react to voices and other sounds from outside the womb. Dr. Lewis Lipsitt, director of the Child Study Center at Brown University, has observed, "It's a threshold area of research, but the data are unequivocal in demonstrating that the fetus hears and feels and has taste."[1]

Other researchers have proved that the unborn child responds to touch, light, and sound. Dr. Michele Clements in London discovered that sixteen-week-old babies became calm when Mozart was played, but kicked violently when they were subjected to rock music.

Dr. Jacob Steiner at the Child Study Center experimented with fetus taste preferences. He noted, "Babies, before they have ever eaten, show a preference for the sweet taste. And it can't be that they prefer it five minutes after they are born and haven't preferred it before."[2] Steiner also tested the babies' sense of smell, using fish, rotten eggs, vanilla, bananas, and strawberries. The babies clearly preferred the pleasant odors. Research also indicates that a baby can recognize his mother's smell.

In 1980 researchers at the University of North Carolina tested hearing and learning abilities to attempt to discover if infants recognize their mothers' voices. The research confirmed their suspicions that they did. Flo McDaniel, director of the American College of Nurse Midwives in Washington, D.C., notes, "What all this means is that you can bond, you can form an attachment to a baby before birth because that baby responds. And every mother, knowing that this baby can be stimulated, should be careful about what she puts into her body. If you get drunk, that baby is going to feel it."[3]

A child can be traumatized by his parents before he is even born. I am familiar with one case in which a child began crying within minutes after birth when she heard her father's voice. As the parents were interviewed, they admitted that they had had some furious arguments during the pregnancy. This unfortunate child came into the world afraid of her own father, learning to fear his voice while she was still inside her mother's womb.

There is ample evidence that a woman can impair her child's health by failing to maintain a good diet or by engaging in harmful activities such as smoking, drinking alcohol, or taking drugs. A certain heroin addict gave birth to her first son while she was in prison. To no one's surprise, her son was born a heroin addict and endured withdrawal symptoms. Happily, he is doing fine today. If this woman had not received medical help, her son might have remained a heroin addict.

The evidence is clear, therefore, that mothers and fathers are teaching and molding their children even in the womb. Expectant parents are wise to cultivate a loving relationship during pregnancy and use their time together to reinforce their love. This helps not only to prepare the mother for childbirth, but also to prepare the unborn subconsciously to identify with both males and females. Since they can distinguish high and low sounds, they doubtless are able to differentiate the voices of their mothers and fathers. An unborn exposed only to loving tones and conversations between his parents will be preprogrammed to think well of both sexes.

If a child can be traumatized against one of the sexes, by quarreling or worse, even before birth, how much will this affect his self-esteem, sexual orientation, and acceptance of his sexual identity? Experts agree that children thrive in a loving environment after birth. I believe they benefit from such an environment even before birth.

THE WONDER OF LEARNING

God has instilled children with a great capacity to learn about the world around them while they are still in the womb. Research has demonstrated that the child begins to learn almost from the moment his brain and nervous system have developed.

Experts in child development tell us that the most important period of development is infancy through age four. Scientists estimate that at least one-half of a child's intellectual capacity has been reached by the fifth year, and 80 percent by the age of eight. This refers to the intelligence level, not to the amount of information the child's mind receives.

During a child's first three months of life, he must have seven basic needs supplied in abundance by a loving mother and father. He must be regularly fed, kept warm, afforded plenty of sleep, cuddled and stroked, given bodily exercise, changed regularly, and provided with sensory and intellectual stimulation.

At the moment we first hold a wrinkly new baby in our arms, we inaugurate a sex-education program. We are teaching the baby about love and warmth and comfort—three essential elements in developing close relationships.

Unlike animals, which are able to take care of many of their own needs fairly soon after birth, a human being is born into this world totally helpless. God has made him totally dependent on other people for every physical and emotional need.

Dr. George E. Gardner, a Boston children's psychiatrist, has observed that relating to other humans is the most important facet of a child's development during the early years. He says, "It is the beginning of all the experiences that depend upon a positive feeling of love, affection, and trust toward other human beings. . . . The many pleasurable experiences the infant has very early in life with his own mother, or the one person who is responsible for his care, generate these feelings of trust and security. . . . From his mother he learns to trust others."[4]

From birth through the third year, a child is dependent primarily on his mother—for such qualities as praise and comfort as well as feeding and diaper changing. During this period a child develops a fear of strangers and clings tenaciously to his mother. God designed the mother's breast purposely so that an infant must be held and caressed to be fed. Emotional security gained during feeding is as important to the infant as the nutrition from mother's milk. Somehow the mother is communicating her love to her dependent child every time she nurses him.

To the benefit of this generation, breast feeding has returned to popularity. At the time my own children were born it was thought old-fashioned to nurse. Manufactured formula was a substitute for mother's milk, so babies were weaned as quickly as possible and put on "the bottle." Bottles, nipples, and formula may have been good for the economy, but it did nothing for a baby's emotions. Some years ago I wrote a book entitled *How to Win Over Depression** in which I predicted that twenty years of bottle-feeding children would soon produce a society of adults with the highest depression rate in the history of mankind. Today we

---

*Grand Rapids: Zondervan, 1974.

have a suicide rate down into the junior high school level that is cause for national alarm.

Children who feel unloved will have a higher rate of depression and attempted suicide than children who in infancy enjoy the emotional security of being nestled next to their mother's body while they are fed. Because the return-to-nature movement has popularized doing the natural in contrast to the synthetic, more mothers than ever are breast feeding their children. Not only does a baby benefit, but mothers testify that they too enjoy the feelings aroused by such a clinging and dependent little life.

Mother is the principle sex-education teacher during the first three years of life. But modern research suggests that a father has a much more significant influence on his child sexually than was believed earlier. It is often from the father that a child gains his or her sex direction.

WHAT IS NORMAL?

The press, liberal educators, and some equally liberal sociologists have almost intimidated our nation against openly and honestly facing the issue of "normal" and "abnormal" sexual behavior. The Christian community sees the issue in true perspective because the Bible is so clear on the subject. One view is called natural, the other "an abomination" or a perversion.

Normal sexuality is the direction that is right for you. That is determined by your sexual apparatus. The problem is, the brain is the most important sex organ in any human being and, much like a computer, the brain is influenced by the data put into it. This is why it is important that infant and early childhood training be provided by both father and mother. As we have seen, a mother is the principle teacher in early childhood, but a father's presence in a loving way is very significant to the young child in developing the right mental images of sexuality and particularly sex direction.

When a father accepts and loves his child, including his sexual identity, it is much easier for the child to accept his natural sex direction at puberty. These impressions are made at an early age.

Most homosexuals claim they were "born that way." In fairness to them, we can say that they probably think this is the case because they cannot recall having any heterosexual feelings. As far back as they can remember, their feelings were homosexual; consequently, they conclude they were born that way. The truth is, they were led that way unintentionally by the influence of one or both parents.

Dr. George A. Rekers, head of the Department of Family and Child Development at Kansas State University, believes that children raised without a father are more likely to have feminine characteristics and become homosexual than those raised with a loving father in the home.

One study found that young boys whose fathers were absent from the home were more likely to exhibit more feminine ways of thinking, low masculinity, dependence, and either less aggression or exaggeratedly masculine behaviors than were boys whose fathers were present. Other studies have also reported negative effects on the sex-role development of boys that are associated with the father's absence. Boys who were separated from their fathers during their preschool years were more often called sissies than were boys who had not been separated from their fathers.

A group of forty-one male orphans who had been reared exclusively by women from six months to five years of age were studied. A battery of psychological tests found these boys to score in the feminine direction as compared with a control group of boys who lived in homes with fathers. When the orphan boys were five years old, half of the group were moved to cottages where a married couple took care of the children. The orphan boys who lived with the father figure later had masculinity scores that were higher than those of the other orphans, who had remained in the totally feminine environment. However, it was found that both groups of orphans still remained relatively low on their masculinity scores as compared with the control group who had fathers present from earliest infancy.

In studies that compare boys with fathers to boys without fathers, the fatherless boys are more likely to be perceived as effeminate than are the boys with fathers. When fatherless boys become adults, they have less successful heterosexual adjustment than do males who grew up in homes with a father. Therefore, all these studies indicate that the absence of the father can have a detrimental effect upon normal heterosexual role development in boys.[5]

This does not mean that boys raised without a father will be homosexuals. I am not suggesting that at all. My own father died when I was nine years old, and my brother was only seven weeks old. Obviously he never knew a father, yet he is definitely heterosexual. I point this out to encourage single mothers who are trying to raise their sons to have normal sexual identities. The odds are that they will.

Even when family lifestyles overexpose children to femininity in the absence of a strong masculine presence, only a small percentage of the children move toward homosexuality. But Dr. Rekers points out that the percentage is higher among those who do not have a loving father figure in their early formative years. Thus the extended family— brothers, grandfathers, uncles, and close church members—can exert a powerful influence on a growing child.

Our emphasis so far has been on the father-son relationship. Infant girls need to observe the role of a loving father also. More will be said about this in the next chapter.

CHILDREN ARE SELFISH

A newborn baby is growing daily in his intellectual abilities. One of the first tasks he must accomplish is to realize that he is separate from his surroundings. During these first exercises of his thinking processes, he comes to the conclusion that he is at the center of everything around him.

A child is naturally born with a concern only for himself. He is instinctively egocentric and selfish. Viewing himself as the center of the universe, the baby—even into toddler-hood—wants his desires satisfied immediately. He has no concept of selflessness or charity. These are moral concepts that must be taught to him if he is to mature into a responsible adult.

Dr. Lawrence Kohlberg, a professor at Harvard University, has written extensively about the various levels of moral development that normally take place as a person grows. Until about ten years of age, Kohlberg says, children are operating on a moral system that is selfish in its orientation. Kohlberg calls this the "concern for self" and identifies two stages at this level: (1) Will I get punished? and (2) What's in it for me?

At the most primitive level, a baby or toddler is largely concerned about whether he will receive punishment for his actions. He knows nothing about "right" and "wrong" and cannot comprehend "sharing" or "giving to others." His world is restricted to satisfying his own needs.

Gardner has pointed out that during the second through fifth years of his life, a child is gaining a moral sense—that is, concepts of right and wrong. "The mechanism of control that we call the 'superego,' which is destined to become unconscious and automatic in its operation, is established."[6] This, says Gardner, is what we call the "conscience," which unconsciously controls our behavior.

PLEASURE AND PAIN

Early in life a child realizes that he will experience two kinds of feelings: pleasure and pain. Accordingly he will elect to try to do things that give him pleasure. After receiving several spankings, he determines that some actions will result in pain. He is learning from his parents the difference between "right" and "wrong" behavior. At this stage of development, the child is incapable of sophisticated reasoning. He learns moral behavior by being rewarded for good behavior (hugs, kisses, loving approval) and by receiving the "rod of correction" for his disobedience.

During his second and third years the child develops a sense of personal identity and gradually learns that he is not the center of the world, but merely part of it. This may cause frustration for him, of course, because he must share his parents' attention with others. At this age he also finds himself in situations where he must interact with peers. Although still egocentric, he will learn how to cope with the requirement that he cooperate rather than make demands.

The development of his ability to use language is a significant turning point in the child's behavior. Parents can now communicate directly and verbally with him on a simple level and administer instructions. The use of verbal commands and the rod will reinforce the parents' moral system on a toddler. As his ability to speak develops, he becomes more sociable and begins to interact with other people.

At the age of two or three the child is a bundle of energy, ceaseless in his quest for new information. He is constantly moving and assimilating what he sees around him.

Until the child has developed the ability to use language, it is impossible to teach him specific information about sex. But a wise mother and father will begin immediately after the birth of their child to teach him about obedience. They will start by distinguishing clearly between good and bad behavior. Because the child is pleasure-oriented and will avoid pain, parents should communicate simple moral values through the "rod of correction." He should learn early that tipping over furniture, biting, throwing toilet water on the floor, and turning on the stove are not acceptable behavior and will be punished.

Parents are responsible to train their pleasure-oriented, independent-minded, and egocentric child to be considerate, self-disciplined, and obedient. This lifelong process cannot begin too early. Using the rod is the appropriate method of controlling the child's behavior and giving him moral training before he is able to speak.

All parental correction, however, must be administered in love. Two key elements must be present in any training of children: love and discipline. A child must know his boundaries; he must understand that certain behavior is acceptable, other actions unacceptable. He must also be made to understand that he will be dealt with consistently, lovingly, and firmly when he crosses the boundaries set for him.

Long before a parent can teach him about sex, a child is already nurturing a sense of morality. As the child learns to speak and respond to his parents' directions, Mom and Dad slowly but surely are developing what will become his "conscience."

Along with moral development during these early years, the child begins to build what Dr. Gardner has called a "hierarchy of values." The child sorts out various objects or people in his little world and decides which are most important to him. Most likely he will choose his mother as his top priority. In second place he will normally select a teddy bear, a blanket, or some other security object.

Security is highly important to a toddler. All manner of fears and anxieties can crush the spirit of a child who finds himself neglected, abused, or shuttled from home to home during these years. Stability is essential if the child is to become a well-adjusted adult.

I find it tragic that day-care centers have become such an important part of American life. Mothers are unaware of the emotional damage they are doing to their children by dropping them off each day while pursuing careers. There is no person in the world who can provide a child with as much love and affection as his natural mother. These children are being deprived of an essential element in their development: mother love. No baby-sitter or child-development specialist can supply the individualized and sincere love that a mother can give her own child. (I realize that single parents must of necessity use the services of day-care centers or baby sitters.

This is one of the unfortunate consequences of the break-down of the American family.) Children are more vulnerable to illness and disease at day-care centers than at home. Evidence is also mounting that child abusers and pornographers are actually opening day-care centers to gain access to innocent children.

ACQUIRING SEXUAL KNOWLEDGE

A two-or-three-year-old will eventually begin to wonder where he came from. If his mother is expecting another child, his curiosity will lead him to ask the first of an endless series of questions about sexual matters. Remember that sex education is a long-term process. A toddler has a short attention span and forgets easily. Most of the time he will assimilate only part of what we say, but we are building his sexual knowledge block by block through the years.

The key to teaching young children is the repetition of information until it becomes ingrained in their thinking. It is a process that begins at birth and lasts until the children leave home. What is important at this stage is to treat a child's questions about sex as casually as we do his questions on any other subject. If we become tense on this issue, he will too. If we treat it as any ordinary subject, so will he.

Toddlers are literalists, that is, they view the world in concrete terms. Their minds have not developed to the point where they can understand symbolism or abstract concepts such as "honor" or "purity." However, they possess the kind of trust and faith that Jesus admired so much (Matthew 18:2–4; 19:14). Unable to reason, they take everything at face value. Usually they will believe anything they are told, so it is very important to be accurate in offering sexual information.

If, for example, a parent says that God placed a seed inside Mommy's tummy, a child will accept that as fact. He will believe that babies grow inside the mother's stomach instead of in the womb. If you have likened the mother's egg to a plant seed, the child will probably visualize a plant growing inside her. At dinnertime he may very well think that the baby "inside your tummy" is being smothered by milk, vegetables, and roast beef!

When talking with our children, we should not enter into a complicated explanation of the reproduction process or sexual intercourse. When he asks a question such as "Where did I come from?" we need not spend an hour explaining everything we know about fetal development. We can simply give him a clear, matter-of-fact answer.

We may also initiate a conversation if we sense that a child has some questions about his origins. To explain sexual reproduction plainly, we can introduce our children to the world of plants, animals, and insects. Watching baby chickens hatch is a good way to inform our children about sex. If a dog or cat is pregnant, we will have an excellent opportunity to explain how God has created life. I have known parents who bought a dog and had her bred so they could teach their children about sex.

I will never forget the time when my three-year-old grandson took me out to the rabbit hutch to explain "why Sugar is so fat." He knew the whole story. He told me how the family took Sugar over to see Thumper. "He is a daddy rabbit. He got Sugar pregnant and now she's going to have some babies." When I asked how soon they would be born, he casually answered, "As soon as she gets big enough."

I was struck by how casual yet intrigued my grandson was about the mystery of life. That's why it is important for us to explain to our children the story of Creation—how God created male and female, plants and animals and insects—and how everything He made was "good." God fashioned every living creature with seeds inside it to reproduce itself. Apples from apple seeds, chickens from eggs, butterflies from eggs that first turn into caterpillars, kittens from within the mother cat.

It may be helpful to convey concrete information to our

children by using drawings to show how God has given living creatures several different ways of creating new living things.

BISEXUAL REPRODUCTION

If you have forgotten some of the information you were taught in high school biology class, here is an elementary lesson in reproduction. This information is provided for you to use as you see fit in explaining sexuality to your children.

Bisexual Reproduction

God has introduced both **asexual** *and* **bisexual** *reproduction in our world. In asexual reproduction, an organism splits in half and becomes two identical objects. Microscopic, one-celled organisms reproduce in this manner. Plants like the hydra propagate themselves in this way by "budding"; a small portion of the plant simply falls off and begins to grow on its own.*

A mother and father are involved in bisexual reproduction. The mother's egg and the father's sperm have to join together. When these two cells merge, the egg is fertilized and a baby begins to grow. God has created three different ways for this to happen: (1) Fertilization can take place outside the mother's body. With fish, for example, the female lays eggs on the bottom of the river; the male swims to them, releases his sperm over them, and swims away; (2) An egg can be fertilized inside the mother's body but develops outside it. This is how chicks are born. The rooster places his sperm inside the chicken to fertilize the egg; the egg then develops a shell around it, and the chicken lays the egg. By keeping the eggs warm, the mother hen helps her baby chicks to mature inside the shell until it is time for them to peck their way out of the egg; (3) The male can fertilize the egg inside the mother, and the baby grows inside until it is ready to be born. Dogs, cats, elephants, horses, and human beings all bear offspring in this way.

TEACHING A TODDLER ABOUT SEX

The teaching lessons may last no longer than five minutes, but we will gradually be building an understanding of sexual matters in our children. Month by month, as the children grow, we can impart more information.

If we choose to equip our toddlers with sexual information, we should familiarize them with words like *penis, vagina, vulva, ova, and sperm.* In discussing sexual matters with our children, we should use the correct medical terms even though we might feel uneasy at first. But if we teach ourselves to refer to the sex organs as casually as we do other parts of the body, we will soon feel comfortable in dealing with this subject. We use correct terms for all other parts of the body, so why should we not be as accurate in describing sexual parts? The important thing for our children's well-being is to be accurate and natural about it.

Toddlers will eventually want to know the names of their sex organs. When a boy asks about his genitals ("What is this?"), give a matter-of-fact answer: "It's your penis. God made all boys to have penises and when boys grow into men they have larger penises." For a girl, answer, "That's a part of your body called the labia. It is two flaps of skin that help to keep germs out of the part of your body where your urine comes from."

At ages two and three, the typical youngster is looking for simple answers to questions. For instance, if he asks, "Where did I come from?" I suggest this answer: "You grew within a small bag inside your mommy, just below her tummy. When you were big enough to be born, you came out through an opening between mommy's legs called the vagina."

If he asks, "How did I get inside your body?" you can answer, "When God created mommies and daddies, he put tiny eggs inside each of us. The daddy has what is called sperm inside his body, and the mommy has tiny eggs. When the sperm from the daddy meets with the egg inside the mommy, a little baby begins to grow in a bag just below mommy's tummy called the uterus."

What if a toddler asks how the sperm gets inside the mommy? I don't think it is necessary to explain sexual intercourse to two-or-three-year-olds. It may not traumatize them, but it could lead to confusion and an unhealthy preoccupation with a mature matter. We can simply promise to tell the child more when he is a little bit older. That will normally satisfy his curiosity.

If a child wonders, "Why does Mommy have to go to the hospital to have a baby?" a suitable answer is, "She must go to the hospital so the doctors can help her give birth to the baby. The doctors will make sure Mommy is comfortable and that the baby is born healthy."

"Why does Mommy have big breasts?" Answer: "All grown-up women have large breasts. God made women this way because a mommy's breasts will fill up with milk when she has a baby. This milk is food for the baby until it is old enough to take milk from a bottle or eat regular food."

"Can any man and woman have babies?" Answer: "Yes, they can, but God wants only men and women who are married to have babies. He wants every baby to have a safe home, where it is loved and cared for by a mother and father."

By the age of three, toddlers should have simplistic knowledge of how babies are born. They should have a general idea of how babies are made, have positive feelings about their own sex, and have a warm, trusting relationship with both mother and father. As children grow older, they will probably ask the same questions over again. Each time we can provide more detailed answers.

A Christian psychologist has noted, "Good sex education begins with your attitudes, depends on the accuracy of your information, and is learned only in an atmosphere of responsibility."[7]

3

Preschool—Ages Four and Five

AT AGES FOUR and five a normal child will develop the ability to use reason in coping with his world. Instead of merely reacting to his environment as he did as a toddler, he will begin to think about the world around him—and question everything. He will gradually identify a cause-and-effect relationship in his environment.

The preschooler's developing language abilities will enable him to learn about the seemingly endless array of objects, places, and people in his new world. Being able now to put thoughts into words, he will begin a lifelong quest for knowledge and understanding. If he is a typical child, he will probably get on his parents' nerves with incessant questioning: Why does the sun shine? Why is the grass green? How do birds fly? As he matures, he will invariably ask where babies come from.

During these three years a child is mastering language, elementary thinking processes, and a concept of selfhood. In addition, he is developing a conscience, a moral sense of right and wrong. Dr. Selma Fraiberg, writing in *The Magic Years,* discusses the formation of the conscience: "Such a conscience does not emerge in the child until the fifth or sixth year. It will not become a stable part of his personality until the ninth or tenth year. It will not become completely independent of outside authority until the child becomes independent of his parents in the last phase of adolescence."[1]

Depending on the kind of training we provide for our children, they will begin to form a distinctive sense of morality. As we teach them about sex, it is absolutely essential that we include sound biblical principles of morality in our discussion. Explaining reproduction without including a moral foundation will prove disastrous. We will deal with sexual morality in greater detail later.

The preschool child is becoming a social person. He enjoys playing with other children and learns to give and take when placed in a social situation. By age five he becomes aware of his own "personhood" and value. He is gaining in self-respect and is developing a sense of self-sufficiency. He enjoys doing things for himself and feels good about his accomplishments.

Dr. George E. Gardner calls this stage of development the period of "romantic learning." The child is anxious to discover everything he can about the world around him. He usually is not learning out of selfish reasons or personal gain, however; he desires to learn simply for the joy of gaining knowledge. Upon entering school he will shift to what Gardner calls "precision learning"—studying with a clear purpose or end in view.

The four-to-six-year-old should be gaining a sense of self-discipline and self-control as his conscience develops. Gardner explains that the development of these positive attributes should follow this pattern: (1) The child learns to control his bodily functions; (2) he is able to govern his aggression against others; (3) he gains a sense of property (not everything belongs to him); (4) he learns to control pleasurable drives or fantasies; (5) he is able to check infantile sexual impulses.[2]Not all children experience early sexual impulses, and those who do are not "perverted" or "oversexed." The wise parent will be watchful of his child without reacting—overreacting—as if sexual impulses pose a significant problem. Usually a restrained parental response is appropriate, for the child will soon proceed into the latency period.

Regarding this concept, Dr. Raymond Moore advises in *Better Late Than Early*, "The ultimate goal of behavior is self-control, self-discipline. We do not prepare our children for the realities of life when we are always telling them what to do and what not to do. Rather, we should allow them to use their own judgment more as they grow older, remembering, however, to keep their choices within the limits of their abilities."[3]

LEARNING ABOUT BABIES

During these years a child is intensely interested in gaining the approval of his mother and father. He looks to them as the final authority on every subject. This attitude of receptivity provides an ideal opportunity to begin a graduated program of formal sex education geared to the interest level of the child. Remember to deal with each child as an individual. Not all five-year-olds are ready to accept the same information. In fact, we may find a younger child more receptive to a discussion of sex than an older sibling. (We must also realize that girls typically mature faster than boys. A five-year-old girl is a year or more ahead of a five-year-old boy in emotional and physical development. This difference doesn't level out until the late teenage years.)

How can we decide whether or not our children are willing to talk about sexual matters? One way is to openly suggest that the preschooler sit down and chat with us. Then we must allow his reaction to direct us. We should be careful not to force unwanted information on him at this age. By being sensitive in our communication about sexuality at this stage in a child's life, we lift the taboo and make it easier for our children to ask more crucial questions at the onset of puberty.

In the sex-saturated society in which we live, it is virtually impossible to keep children isolated from pictures, magazines, movies, or television programs that display sex in offensive ways. Cable movie channels often show R-rated movies that contain explicit sex, profanity, and violence. We can only wonder how many children are regularly exposed to sex scenes on television that are far beyond their age level to comprehend and evaluate.

At school our youngsters will be exposed to children who have acquired inaccurate sexual information from objectionable television programming. Older children often show off their sexual knowledge by describing sexual activities to younger, less-informed children.

The point is that our children—especially those in public schools—are going to learn about sex. It is far better that we convey accurate information and correct attitudes under controlled conditions than allow the children to acquire distorted views from their friends. Sex education on the school playground usually comprises a lurid description of sexual intercourse that totally ignores the emotions and commitments connected with it and strips it of its beauty. Our children should never be led to believe that the act of marriage is simply a biological function; rather, it is God's way of joining a husband and wife together in sacred unity.

Our most important asset in teaching our children about sex, love, and marriage is having a healthy attitude about these subjects ourselves. Our mannerisms, tone of voice, and gestures will all convey either positive or negative feelings to our children. If we are still carrying any guilt about sexual matters from childhood, we would be wise to get our own feelings and thoughts in order before beginning to convey sex information to our offspring. A careful reading of *The Act of Marriage* will help to provide a positive attitude toward this subject.

A light-hearted, casual approach to sex education will

remove many of the bad feelings that children might have developed from premature exposure to sexual matters at school. We can let our children know right up front that we are willing to discuss sexual matters. We don't have to reveal everything at once—and we can tell them so.

Dr. James Dobson tells the story of his experience of working with top secret documents in the military service. In his particular area, certain documents were unavailable to him or were given to him only on a "need-to-know" basis. He compares this experience to our procedure in teaching children about sex.

At ages four, five, or six our children do not need to know every last detail of the act of marriage from foreplay to climax. We should reveal this information as they require it. A direct question does not necessitate a detailed answer. If possible, we should respond to explicit questions briefly and to the point without adding details. Usually a straightforward answer will satisfy the questioner. If not, we can tell them that we will be glad to discuss it when they are a little older and that they are free to remind us then.

EXPLAINING FETAL DEVELOPMENT

Where do we begin an explanation about sexual reproduction to our children at the preschool level? A child who wants to know how a baby develops inside the mother can benefit from a simple explanation. With this explanation you may wish to use the diagrams included in this chapter or draw your own pictures to give your children a visual image of this miraculous event.

We might begin with the account of Creation in the Book of Genesis. We recount the story of the Garden of Eden, showing the children that God made both the male and the female, blessed His creation, and told Adam and Eve to multiply and subdue the earth.

Male and Female

God invented two sexes—male and female. He created men and women to love and support each other. He also instituted marriage, wherein a man and woman would marry and live together for the rest of their lives. In this marriage relationship, He expected Adam and Eve to create a family by having children. Within this family, He anticipated that godly parents would love their children and teach them about Himself, the world, and relationships such as sex.

When God directed Adam and Eve to have children, He wanted them to reproduce, to create new lives. He declared that people should populate the whole earth. But how is new life created? We might explain sexual reproduction to the preschooler in these terms:

When God created the world, He made all the insects, plants, animals and people. In every living creature He placed tiny seeds or eggs so that everything that lives can reproduce its kind. A mother cat, for example, has eggs inside her body, and a tomcat has tiny sperm. When the egg from the mother joins the sperm from the father, a baby cat is created and begins to grow slowly inside the mother's body. The baby cat grows in the uterus. (Perhaps we will have the opportunity to show our children the birth of kittens or some other domestic animal. This would be an excellent way to impress these facts on them.)

Human mothers have babies in much the same way as animals. Inside every female are thousands of tiny eggs smaller than the period at the end of this sentence. When one of these eggs meets with a sperm inside the uterus, a new baby is created.

Our bodies are made up of millions of cells, but when a baby is first created, it is only one cell—so small that we can't see it without looking through a microscope. But this cell splits into two cells, then four, continuing to grow and grow. In its early stage, the developing baby is called an **embryo.** *Later in the baby's growth it is called a* **fetus,** *a word that means "young one."*

As the cells begin to multiply, this new baby finds a comfortable place in the soft lining of the uterus and begins to grow. Inside the mother's uterus (which is shaped like an upside-down pear), the baby grows until it is large enough to live outside the mother.

How does the baby eat? He is fed by his mother through a cord attached to his stomach. The other end of this **umbilical cord** *is connected to the wall of the uterus. We can imagine what this is like by thinking of an astronaut walking out in space, attached to the spaceship by a cord. In space there is no air for the astronaut to breathe, so he gets his air through the cord attached to his suit. The baby gets his air and food through the umbilical cord.*

After about nine months, the baby is big enough to be born. The uterus begins to squeeze and squeeze (an action we call **labor contractions**). *Slowly but surely the baby is squeezed out of the uterus and into the vagina and then out of the mother's body.*

A doctor or nurse or midwife helps the mother to give birth to her baby.

As we explain these facts of reproduction to our children, we should make sure to stress the wonder of God's creation. It is important for them to understand that God made them and loves them very much. They should realize that everything in God's creation is good, including sexual reproduction.

CORRECTLY NAMING BODY PARTS

Some parents today fear having to correctly name the sexual organs for their children. As youngsters many parents were

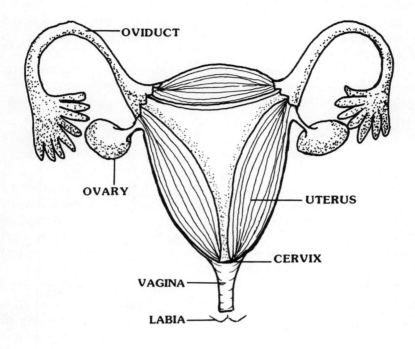

The internal and external female sexual organs.

never given the right names; they somehow sensed that sexual terms and bodily functions were "dirty" or "wrong." Each family had its own euphemisms for urination, defecation, the penis, the vagina, and so on. Unfortunately, this increases the difficulties of communicating healthful attitudes and avoiding negative impressions as parents teach their children about sexuality.

The following terms are identified in the diagrams in this chapter.

Female Organs

Ovaries. Two small containers in the mother's body hold thousands of eggs. Each of these is called an ovary. When an egg leaves the ovary, it travels down a tube toward the uterus where it can meet the sperm.

Oviduct. This is a tube through which an egg travels toward the uterus as it awaits fertilization.

Uterus. The uterus is like a little room where the baby grows inside the mother. This room, shaped like an upside-down pear, is like a balloon—that is, it gets bigger and bigger as the baby grows.

Cervix. This is a passageway between the uterus and the vagina. It is normally no wider than a pencil lead, but it expands during childbirth.

Vagina. When the baby is large enough to be born and come out into the world, it descends from the uterus, enters a tube or tunnel called the vagina, and continues to the outside world. All girls have a vagina, uterus, and eggs. But God designed girls so they can't have children until they are close to being teenagers.

Labia. To protect the vagina from germs, there are two folds of skin, called labia, over the entrance to the vagina. Inside these folds are smaller folds of skin and a sex organ called the clitoris. This area of a girl's body is known as the *vulva.*

Male Organs

Testicles. These organs produce the sperm cells which, when joined to the mother's egg, form a new baby.

Scrotum. This is the bag of skin behind the penis. There are two peanut-shaped organs called testicles inside the scrotum.

Spermatic Duct. This is a main duct through which sperm pass from the scrotum to and through the penis.

Penis. This is the male sex organ. Through this organ sperm cells leave the body, and waste water or urine is released.

As the children grow older, they will need additional and more detailed information about reproduction. This is provided in another chapter.

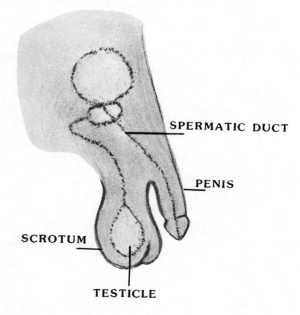

SPERMATIC DUCT

PENIS

SCROTUM

TESTICLE

The male reproductive system.

PARENTAL CONCERNS

Masturbation

Masturbation sometimes becomes a primary concern of parents of four-to-six-year-olds. According to Dr. Clyde Narramore, masturbation is practiced by some children between the ages of two to six and again between the ages of twelve and twenty.

What should parents do if their children masturbate? Narramore advises, "Infrequent acts of masturbation should be ignored. This is not easy to do when one has been taught that masturbation causes all sorts of dreadful things. But try your best to accept the fact that there is no physical basis for being afraid or worried. Your *attitude* will more than likely determine the end results."[4] A child who masturbates is not demonstrating a depraved mind. He is just giving evidence that he has discovered a pleasurable aspect of his body. If he fondles himself in public, a parent should speak to him calmly in private about it, explaining that this should not be done in public. We can be diplomatic; we shouldn't foster negative feelings about the sex organs. But neither should we let a child become an exhibitionist.

A compulsive or chronic practice of masturbation might indicate an emotional difficulty of some kind. Consult a trusted physician if you feel that your child is overly preoccupied with his genitals.

Sex Play

Sex play often alarms parents. When they discover their children involved in coeducational nudity, the normal reaction is anger or indignation. At ages four, five, or six it is quite common for children to satisfy their curiosity by exploring each other's bodies. Playing "doctor" or "nurse" is one of the ways children investigate the anatomy of the opposite sex.

This sex play should be firmly discouraged, but resist the temptation to get angry. By simply telling our children and those involved that this is inappropriate behavior, we should be able to eliminate casual or secretive sex play. We should let the child know that he should learn about male and female differences from us, not from personal investigation. We can help him to realize that our bodies are private and that therefore we are not to expose them to others or touch the private parts of another person.

Sex Roles

Sex roles are a greater concern than they once were. Feminists, humanists, and "sexologists" in our culture are advocating a unisex society where men and women will supposedly dress alike, think alike, and be able to choose sexual lifestyles freely—heterosexual, homosexual, or bisexual. Our children are being bombarded with this propaganda through transvestite rock stars such as Boy George and Prince. We can expect transvestism to become a more serious sexual characteristic in the years ahead as social revolutionaries attempt to confuse sexual roles.

Little boys often dress in their mother's clothing, and girls sometimes don their father's outfits. Before our society was assaulted by sex revolutionaries, this would have been considered harmless play, for children love to put on costumes. Unfortunately, in our day harmless play could lead to sex-role confusion.

If our young children want to play "dress-up," we should encourage our daughters to dress in female clothing and our sons in men's clothes. We should be certain that a clear dividing line exists between male and female dress and personal appearance.

In addition, both mothers and fathers should be reinforcing specific sex roles for their children. In his book *Sex Roles and the Christian Family,* W. Peter Blitchington writes, "During the first five or six years of life, the young child's sexual identity will be formed. A boy needs contact with his father in order for his sexual identity to be developed properly. Boys whose fathers are absent, passive, or rejecting often find it harder to identify with the male role. Overly dominating mothers may also lead a young boy to identify too strongly with his mother and to reject masculinity."[5]

4

Middle Childhood—Ages Six to Ten

IN THEIR BOOK *Child Behavior,* Dr. Frances Ilg and Dr. Louis B. Ames write, "Our observations of child behavior have led us to believe that almost any kind of behavior you can think of (eating, sleeping, talking, moving about, getting on with other people, even thinking about religion or understanding such complicated things as time and space) develops by means of remarkably patterned and largely predictable stages."[1]

Ilg and Ames further explain that every child will go through numerous stages of physical and emotional development as he grows to adulthood. They make no claim that they can predict how a particular child will turn out, but they state that they can pinpoint the different stages he will pass through on his way to maturity.

The "remarkably patterned and largely predictable stages" of child development affirm what the Scriptures say about God's marvelous creation. God has revealed Himself in the patterns and meticulous order of the universe. He has demonstrated to mankind His presence in the orderly and predictable behavior of honey bees; in the changing of the seasons; in the molecular structure of matter. And He has disclosed Himself most clearly in His highest creation: mankind. From the moment of conception through the embryonic and fetal stages to the dramatic hour of delivery, God's hand is strongly evident in the birth of all mankind.

As we teach our children about reproduction and sexual love, we should always make it a point to link these "facts of life" to the existence of an all-powerful, all-loving God. The Bible tells us that "the heavens declare the glory of God" (Psalm 19:1); our conversations with our children should continually emphasize this truth. Our children should come to realize that the process of conception is one of the most miraculous evidences of God's presence and care for His creatures in the universe.

To help you more effectively explain the divinely ordered universe to your children, you may wish to write to the Institute for Creation Research, 2100 Greenfield Drive, El Cajon, California 92021, for a catalog of its various publications and books. We should become well-versed in scientific creationism and then teach our children to view their creation from a biblical perspective. Not only will they have more of a reverence for God's creation, but they will be less likely to succumb to evolutionary theory in school.

ORDERED STAGES OF CHILD BEHAVIOR

From ages six to ten, a typical child is learning to reason, to think things through on his own, and to discern right from wrong behavior. His conscience, or inner control mechanism, is becoming well developed. He is developing the capacity to control his emotions, postpone gratification, and check outbursts of anger when he cannot get his way. The soundness of his values or morals will depend in large measure on our effectiveness as parents in conveying Christian truth. We cannot entrust the moral training of our children to the ungodly or others who do not share our moral values. It is our responsibility to "civilize" our children by teaching them to follow the Lord through our example and through the lessons we teach them from the Word of God.

At age six an average child will readily accept spiritual truths but is not yet able to think in abstract terms. He is a literalist. At seven he is beginning to think abstractly and can better grasp such concepts as "purity," "righteousness," "holiness," and "honor." The eight-year-old will often begin to question teachings that he once accepted on faith. Not a cynic, he is merely eager to discover the truth about spiritual matters. The nine-year-old can be motivated to Christian service through the study of the lives of men and women in the Bible and godly saints who have lived since then. The church of Jesus Christ has produced hundreds of heroes who serve as worthy examples to our children. At ten the child is often ready to discuss why he believes the way he does. He can apply the facts of the Bible to his own life.

During these years a child becomes a social individual, learning to cooperate and interrelate with others—at school, at church, or at play with neighbors. He is beginning to realize that his actions have consequences. He discovers that some behavior is unacceptable and will get him into serious trouble whereas other behavior is affirmed and will be rewarded. He looks to adults for approval. By age seven the child is becoming a well-adjusted member of society, wanting to interact with others. At eight and nine he will join clubs (with members usually being only of his own sex) and participate in group activities (again, his own sex). By age ten segregation between boys and girls is the norm, but only temporarily. Within a few years, at puberty, the opposite sex will suddenly become an obsession.

At age six, children normally display an awareness of and interest in the physical differences between boys and girls. As previously pointed out, they may sometimes play "doctor" or "nurse" in order to explore the bodies of the opposite sex. There may be episodes of sex play or instances in which boys and girls will agree to show each other their genitals to satisfy their curiosity. Naturally this kind of behavior should be discouraged. But we should beware of making a bigger issue out of it than is necessary. We should make it clear to our children, without being severe, that only doctors or parents are allowed to see them in the nude. If necessary, we can satisfy our children's curiosity by showing them drawings of male and female organs.

Seven-year-olds show less interest in sex, but some exploration still takes place. From ages eight to ten, children normally look at sex and elimination as a source of crude jokes. At nine they will begin to talk about sex with their friends and use sexual terms in swearing or in creating poetry. They will be fascinated to learn about their own sex organs.

By age ten most girls and some boys have learned from their friends about menstruation and sexual intercourse—if we haven't already informed them. A wise parent will share this information briefly by the eighth or ninth year to ensure his child's having accurate information. It is far better that details of sexual reproduction come from parents rather than from bathroom walls or misinformed friends.

What are children aged six to ten interested in knowing about sexual reproduction? They are normally curious about conception and the process by which a baby grows inside the mother's body. Many will also inquire about the role of the father in conceiving the child.

THE BEGINNINGS OF LIFE

When God created this world, He fashioned all manner of life forms. He created bugs, bats, fish, turtles, hamsters, ele-phants, birds, and thousands of different kinds of plants. His crowning creation was man and woman. The Book of Genesis tells us that God created every creature with the ability to reproduce itself, or create new life from within its own body. Within every plant are the seeds to create new plants. Within the bodies of animals and humans God designed what we

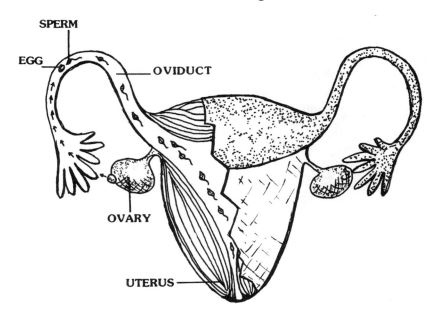

Fertilization in the female's body.

call a *reproductive system* so that each animal and human can create more life.

The sexes have different reproductive systems that complement each other for the propagation of new life. Two males cannot conceive babies, nor can two females. In mammals life can be created only when the sperm from the male joins with the egg from the female. A male has millions of sperm cells; a female has thousands of eggs.

When a sperm cell meets an egg cell, it pushes its way inside. When this happens, we say that the egg has been *fertilized.* This is also called the moment of *conception* because a new baby has just been created. The fertilized egg begins to divide or separate into two cells. Then those two tiny cells split into four and so on until there are far too many cells to count. In the case of a human being, this process continues for nine months until the baby is ready to be born.

Inside the sperm cell and the egg are tiny objects called

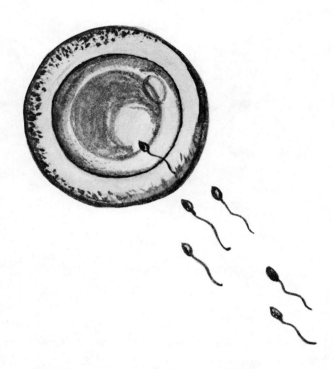

Fertilization of a female's egg by a male's sperm.

chromosomes. Under a powerful microscope these chromosomes look like little bits of string. On the chromosomes are *genes,* which determine what the child is going to look like: his hair and eye color, intelligence, physical abilities, body build and height, temperament and more—in other words, every physical and mental characteristic of the person.

Sperm cells and eggs contain twenty-three chromosomes apiece. When they join together in conception, therefore, there are forty-six. Within each set of chromosomes are fifteen thousand genes. Scientists who study how human life begins have discovered that at least 16 million different combinations could be made in creating a baby. That is, every child that was ever born had the potential to be

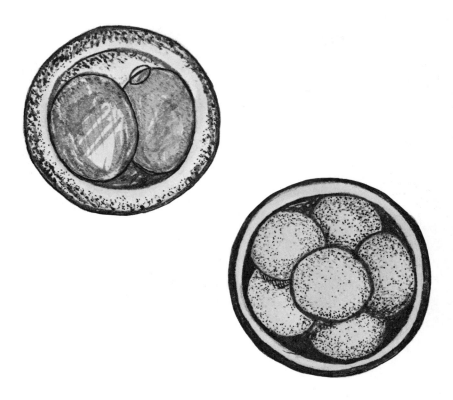

(Top) A fertilized egg when it has divided after thirty hours. (Bottom) The developing embryo after two days.

different in 16 million different ways! With that many choices, it is easy to understand why no two human beings are exactly alike. Even identical twins register different fingerprints, different temperaments, and perhaps contrasting ways of thinking. So every human—in fact, every creation of God—is unique.

In explaining chromosomes and genes to our children, we can compare genes to the instruction booklet we receive with a new bicycle. Upon opening the carton, we pull out all the different parts and then begin to read the instruction booklet to learn how to put the bicycle together. The instruction booklet provides a step-by-step plan for successfully assembling the machine. Without instructions we would have a difficult time making any sense of the various bicycle parts. The same holds true within a male's sperm cell and a female's egg. The genes act as little instruction booklets, forming a blueprint as to how a baby will look and how he will think, his creative tendencies, and of course his temperament, which has a profound effect on his personality and spontaneous actions.

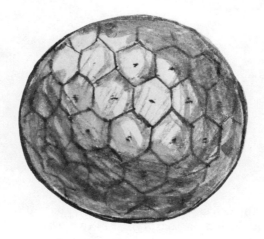

The developing embryo after four days.

A BABY BEGINS TO GROW

The following explanation of conception and development can either be read to children or rephrased in your own words. The illustrations in this chapter will be helpful.

A Baby Begins to Grow

A mother's egg is usually fertilized by the sperm inside a tube in the mother's body known as the **Fallopian tube**. *This is like a short rubbery pipe that leads from the mother's ovaries, where the eggs are kept, down into the uterus, where the baby will grow. Every woman has approximately 400,000 eggs in her ovaries, but only 300 to 400 of them pass out of the ovaries and into the uterus during a woman's lifetime.*

After growing for a few days, the fertilized egg attaches itself to the side of the uterus and begins to develop into a baby. To help the baby mature, a special organ called the **placenta** *grows on the inner wall of the uterus. This is made up of many, many blood vessels that help to feed the baby. Connecting the placenta to the baby's stomach is a long tube called the* **umbilical cord**. *Through this cord the baby receives his food and oxygen via the mother's bloodstream. The baby's waste also passes through this cord into the mother's body; her liver and kidneys will dispose of these waste products. The placenta also acts as a barrier protecting the baby from many harmful substances that might travel in the mother's bloodstream.*

During the second week a special protective covering surrounds the baby as he grows in the uterus. Called the **amniotic sac**, *this covering is filled with a watery substance called* **amniotic fluid**. *This fluid protects the baby from being injured in the uterus and also helps to keep him warm at all times, even when it is freezing outside. In this dark, warm, protected nest the baby grows for nine months until he is ready to be born.*

The Growth Stages of a Baby

At conception a new baby is smaller than the dot of an i. *Within six to twelve hours the fertilized egg divides into two cells, and these continue to divide. Within two months the*

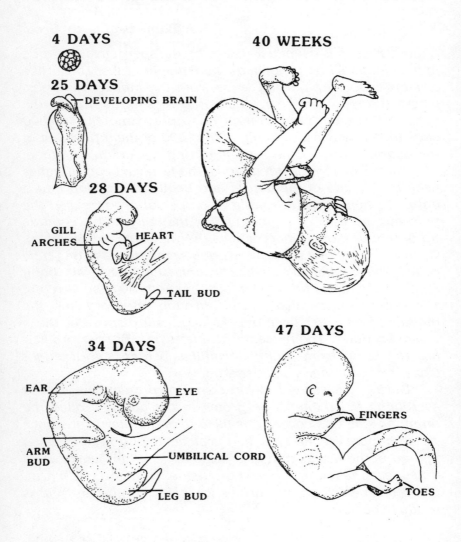

4 DAYS

25 DAYS
DEVELOPING BRAIN

28 DAYS
GILL ARCHES
HEART
TAIL BUD

40 WEEKS

34 DAYS
EAR
EYE
ARM BUD
UMBILICAL CORD
LEG BUD

47 DAYS
FINGERS
TOES

(Counterclockwise from top left) The progress of development of an embryo into a fetus (one month old) and to full term (forty weeks, or nine months).

baby has grown to 240 times his original size and a million times heavier than his original weight as one cell. A newborn baby has millions of cells; an adult has 60 trillion.

When the baby is about five days old, the cluster of cells resembles a berry. This stage of development is called a **morula,** *derived from the Latin word for mulberry. As the morula continues to grow, the cells begin to take on different jobs in forming the baby. Some cells become part of the brain; others become muscle tissue and nerve endings. Still other cells join together to form the eyeballs, ears, nose, mouth, hands, and sexual organs. Through a mysterious process, called* **differentiation,** *that scientists still haven't figured out, each cell knows exactly where to go and what part of the body to become.*

In the first month of life, the **embryo,** *a Greek word meaning "to swell") is about the size of an apple seed. The baby already has a heart, and the brain is beginning to form. The backbone, spinal column, and nervous system are also developing at this time. New scientific research is demonstrating that even from this early stage of development, the embryo is a real, living person.*

In the second month, the brain has formed. Ears, eyes, nose, lips and tongue are taking shape. At this point the baby is called a **fetus,** *a Latin term for "young one" or "offspring." By month's end, all the baby's features are in place. By the ninth week, the fetus has a reproductive system, and thus the baby could be clearly identified as a girl or a boy.*

By the third month the baby, more than two inches in length, develops fingernails and toenails. During the fourth month, eyebrows and eyelashes form, and the baby will suck his thumb for the first time.

In the fifth and sixth months the fetus develops nostrils, and the ears begin to function. The growing baby can hear his mother's voice and can even open his eyes and see. During the seventh through ninth months the baby completes the final stages of development before birth. In his booklet When You Were Formed in Secret, *Gary Bergel describes these final months:*

The skin of the infant thickens and begins to look polished. A layer of fat is produced and stored beneath the skin, both for insulation and as a food supply. Antibodies that give immunity to diseases are built up. A gallon per day of amniotic fluid is absorbed by the baby and the fluid is totally replaced every three hours. The baby's heart now pumps three hundred gallons of blood per day and the placenta begins to age.

Approximately one week before the two hundred and sixtieth day the infant stops growing and "drops," usually head downward, into the pelvic cavity. All preparations are finished and both the mother and child can but wait for the drama of birth.[2]

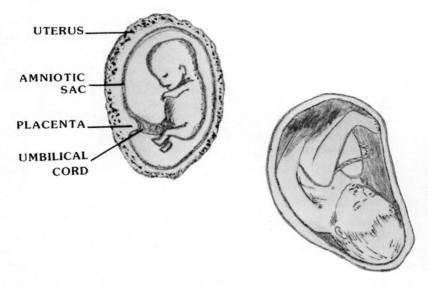

UTERUS

AMNIOTIC SAC

PLACENTA

UMBILICAL CORD

(Left) The fetus protected within the uterus. (Right) The baby in position for birth, which usually happens head first.

The Baby Is Born

No one is really sure how the baby knows when it is time for his passage to the outside world, but the typical human baby is born nine months after conception. The uterus, which is the largest and most powerful muscle in the mother's body, begins to squeeze together to push the baby down through the bottom of the uterus, through an opening called the **cervix** *and into the birth canal, the vagina, and out into the world.*

Usually before the baby is born, the mother knows it is time to go to the hospital, because the amniotic sac breaks open and the fluid flows out of the mother's body. When the mother's "water breaks," as this is called, it is important that she reach the hospital as rapidly as possible to protect the baby. The amniotic sac and fluid are protections for the baby, but when the water is gone, the baby must be delivered quickly. Most doctors prefer that the mother reaches the hospital before this sac is broken.

When the mother is taken into the operating room, the doctors and nurses help her deliver the baby. She often has to push to get the baby to come out through the vagina. A baby is usually born headfirst, and sometimes when he comes through the cervix, his head is squeezed. But God has created the baby's skull with a series of interlocking bones that can be pushed together. Several days after the baby is born, his head is back to a normal shape, and the process does no harm to his brain.

At the moment of birth, when the baby is outside the mother's body, he is still attached to the placenta by the umbilical cord. The doctor cuts off the cord, leaving a small stub. After a few days this stub dries up and falls off. The abdominal area where the umbilical cord was attached to the baby is called the **navel** *or, more commonly, the "belly button."*

TEACHING ABOUT MENSTRUATION AND INTERCOURSE

For most parents, information about sexual intercourse or the menstrual cycle is the most difficult aspect of reproduction to communicate to children. The reasons for parental reluctance vary. Many parents never received proper sex education in their own homes and have never felt comfortable discussing the subject themselves. If it was taboo when they were young, they are likely to be reticent to deal with the subject as adults. In addition, the act of marriage and menstruation are two very personal issues, seldom or never discussed except between spouses. A third reason may be that parents are worried about traumatizing their youngsters with images of "making love" or with fearful thoughts of "bleeding" when the menstrual cycle begins.

How should parents approach these issues? In discussing sexual intercourse, we can first describe sexual reproduction among animals, then lead into a discussion of how mothers and fathers create new life. The following explanation builds on the discussion of reproduction included in the previous chapter.

Sexual Intercourse

In warm-blooded animals such as elephants, horses, dogs, cats, and hamsters, God has equipped the male with a penis. During a certain time of the year, male and female animals **mate** *or have* **sexual intercourse** *with each other. In the case of dogs and cats, for example, this is the time of the year when they are "in heat." When a male and female dog is in heat, the male dog places his penis inside the female dog's vagina and they mate. The sperm from the dog enters the female's body and meets with the egg, creating a puppy. Usually a female dog has several puppies, which we call a litter, and it takes only a few months for these puppies to become fully developed in the mother's womb.*

All animals mate by **instinct,** *which means that they do things without even thinking about them. No animals can think like a human being. They don't even know they exist, but God has put instructions in their brains telling them* when to mate, how to find food, how to protect themselves from enemies, how to build their homes—everything they need to live and survive.

In the animal kingdom, females are able to have babies only during certain times of the year. When their eggs are ready to be fertilized, the females will give off a scent or act in a certain way that is attractive to males. For example, the female tiger in heat will sound a **mating call** to attract a male. If more than one male arrives on the scene, they will fight over the female, and the loser will run away. Wild animals such as tigers and tame animals such as cats mate in much the same way with the same kinds of rituals. For example, after a male tiger has run off any rivals for his mate, the male and female tigers will gently kiss, allowing their whiskers to touch. The female rolls over and plays. After a time, she presents herself to the male, and they engage in sexual intercourse.

All the reproduction that takes place among animals, insects, fish, and birds is the result of instincts that God has programmed into the bodies of these creatures. As the Great Computer Programmer of Living Creatures, God has put all the information needed for survival into the brains (the computers) of all His creatures. Thus, animals do not really think the same way humans do; they merely carry out the directions or instructions God has given them.

Unlike animals, we humans use our brains to reason. Admittedly, we possess certain instincts for survival including automatic reactions when we find ourselves in danger. But God has also given us a free will and the ability to reason. Free will means that we have the freedom and ability to choose how we are going to live. Having granted us the capacity to differentiate between good and evil, God would prefer that we elect to obey Him. By using our God-given reasoning powers, we are aware that we exist; moreover, we have an understanding of the past and present and can plan for the future. We can also use our minds to create useful objects such as televisions, cars, and houses.

An important part of God's plan for mankind is repro-duction—bearing children to carry on the human race. He wants men and women to have children, but only if they are married and have committed themselves to raising these children within the family. God condemns sexual intercourse outside of marriage as a sin. Unfortunately, many people who do not know God choose to mate without being married.

When a husband and wife love each other very much and want to have a baby, they go to bed, hug each other closely, and kiss. During this time of hugging and kissing, the husband will place his penis inside his wife's vagina. When sperm come out of the man's penis, they travel up into the Fallopian tubes. If one sperm cell meets an egg, conception occurs. This is how babies are made. Nine months after conception, a beautiful chubby baby is born—the result of a mom and dad's love for each other.

MENSTRUATION

For an undetermined reason, girls in America are experienc-ing their first periods at an increasingly earlier age. Some theorize that it might be our improved diet, or it might be that more of our population lives in warmer sections of the country. No one has yet provided a satisfactory explanation. But it is known that girls living closer to the equator tend to begin menstruating earlier than those raised in colder climates. Some girls as young as nine years of age begin to menstruate. The following information is essential in prepar-ing girls for this momentous event.

Menstruation

*Deep inside a woman's body are two **ovaries** where the body stores eggs, or **ova**. Each month, when a girl or woman experiences her period, one egg is released from the ovary* *and travels down her Fallopian tube in preparation to meet a sperm cell. Likewise, every month, the woman's uterus gets prepared to hold a fertilized egg approximately seventy-two hours, during which time she is called **fertile**. At this time she can become pregnant, that is, conceive a baby. But most of the time the egg is not fertilized by a sperm; it simply disintegrates or falls apart and leaves the woman's body through her vagina.*

When the uterus prepares to receive the fertilized egg, its lining becomes thick with many blood veins. If a fertilized egg attached itself to the side of the uterus, these veins would be ready to begin providing food for the developing baby. But when no fertilized cell appears, this lining falls apart and is discarded by the woman's body.

*For several days during a month, this thick lining is flowing out of the woman's body. Called a **menstrual flow**, it happens to a woman whether she is married or not. God has equipped every woman with the ability to have children, although not all women choose to get married or have babies. The menstrual flow is commonly called a **period**, and it occurs as a monthly event until a woman reaches forty-five or fifty years of age. To catch this menstrual flow, women use sanitary napkins or tampons.*

Menstruation should be explained by her mother at about a girl's eighth birthday. It does an injustice to a girl not to convey these truths before she experiences her first period. She should be reassured that this is a perfectly natural occurrence, a sign that she is becoming mature enough to bear children. She should also understand that there is nothing "unclean" or "filthy" about her monthly period. And since there are 9 percent more women on earth than men, the majority of the world's population have periods at some time in their lives.

TELLING THE SIMPLE TRUTH

If we deal with these matters of sexual reproduction and menstruation with a relaxed attitude, our children will accept the information we give them without being upset or thinking sex is somehow a dirty secret. By emphasizing God's role in designing this creative process, we will show our children that sex is a wholesome and positive aspect of their lives.

5

Preadolescence—Ages Eleven to Thirteen

IN THE MOVIE *Star Trek—The Search for Spock,* Captain Kirk and the crew of the *Starship Enterprise* search for the spirit of Mr. Spock, who sacrificed his life to save them in a previous Star Trek episode. Spock's casket was launched into space and landed safely on a nearby planet where a group of scientists are attempting to create new life.

When Captain Kirk and his men discover Spock's casket, they find it empty. Instead, they find a Vulcan boy who faintly resembles Spock. To their amazement this boy begins to change and grow before their eyes. In an unusual growth spurt, filled with cries of agony and pain, this preadolescent boy undergoes a miraculous transformation. Within hours the frightened boy becomes a grown man.

Looking back on my own preadolescent years, it seems to me that it would have been far easier to endure several hours of agony and become fully mature like Mr. Spock than to battle ever-changing emotions and physical changes over a period of years. But the Lord didn't make us that way, so we have to learn to adjust to the way things are. What the young Vulcan boy supposedly experienced in a few hours requires years in real life. The emotional changes are sometimes agonizing, but the trauma of preadolescence can be tempered if both parents and children understand what is happening.

Adolescence is that time in a person's life when he is changing from a child into an adult. It is a period that roughly parallels the teenage years, but sometimes begins as early as nine years old in girls. The beginning of adolescence is known as *puberty*. This stage of development is characterized by the maturing of the sexual organs in preparation for reproduction—menstruation in girls and the first presence of sperm in boys—as well as secondary sex characteristics such as pubic hair, underarm hair, enlarged breasts in girls, and deepened voices in boys.

IS YOUR CHILD PUBERTY-STRICKEN?

"Puberty" comes from Latin words referring to "grown-up," "adulthood," "groin," and "body hair." It signifies a definite physical and emotional change in a person, moving him from childhood into adulthood. Puberty can be especially disturbing for boys and girls who have not been properly prepared for it by their parents. Just imagine how horrible it would be if your daughter were sitting in a classroom and she experienced *menarche*—the beginning of menstruation—but hadn't been prepared for it. How well would we cope with that situation if we thought we were bleeding to death in front of our friends? Or imagine the guilt and fear a son would experience after waking to find his sheets soiled with semen if he had not been told about "wet dreams."

We should not put off telling our children about sexual matters if they are near puberty. A little knowledge will go a long way in protecting them from unnecessary trauma. Going through puberty or preadolescence is difficult even when a person has been informed what to expect.

Sex education from parents can almost never be too early. If information is too advanced and technical, it will simply go over the children's heads. But if we are going to get to them before someone who may not share our moral values or sensitivity, we had better start early.

In the previous chapter I dealt with menstruation because many girls experience it as young as nine years of age. In general we will have to tell girls the facts of life earlier than boys. Boys do not usually reach puberty until around age eleven, normally one to two years later than girls.

As our children enter puberty and adolescence, we will face some new and unique challenges. The little ones we once cradled in our arms are now blossoming into adults and are beginning to show adultlike thinking on some occasions. But we will discover quickly that preadolescents vacillate between childlike thinking and adult reasoning. Conflicts are inevitable. We must be ready for them; this is a normal stage of life. Adolescence is also a time when our children begin to pull away from us to establish their independence and a healthful sense of identity.

As parents of children entering puberty we will learn what our parents had to endure as we went through it. We will find out why our parents acted as they did when we were struggling with the emotional ups and downs of adolescence. We will develop our own ways of handling our puberty-stricken children, but we will also gain a better appreciation of our own parents.

What are the various stages our children will experience as they pass through preadolescence toward adulthood? During our children's puberty we will notice not only the obvious physical changes, but changes in attitudes and behavior also. We will discover that the latter are not necessarily positive.

Puberty begins with significant hormonal changes in the body of a boy or girl. Every body has its own internal mechanism for determining when puberty starts, and this moment differs with each child. Puberty can start as early as age nine, as has been stated, but also as late as age sixteen. There is no "right" time chronologically for a child to enter puberty; it depends on the individual's makeup. As already noted, puberty begins earlier in warm climates; but it is delayed when children have poor nutrition.

The onset of puberty is governed by the *endocrine system,* which comprises several glands, including the hypothalamus, the pituitary, the thyroid, the parathyroid, the adrenal glands, and the ovaries or testicles. All these work together to bring about physical and emotional changes in girls and boys.

In a boy the hypothalamus signals the pituitary gland, which in turn releases three key hormones, the *androgens.* These hormones give the boy his masculine qualities, both physical and emotional. The male hormones stimulate aggressiveness, ambition, and drive. (For a more detailed discussion of sex hormones and their effects on masculinity or femininity, I recommend W. Peter Blitchington's book, *Sex Roles and the Christian Family.*)

The three hormones released by the pituitary stimulate the adrenal glands and cause a boy's testicles to begin producing the hormone *testosterone,* the most potent of the male hormones. Testosterone induces the production of sperm cells and the growth of body hair. In addition, the boy's voice box or larynx grows and his voice deepens. Boys may also experience a temporary enlargement of the breasts during puberty. This enlargement is called "gynecomastia" and can sometimes be painful, but is a normal occurrence and should not be cause for alarm.

In a girl the pituitary gland stimulates the production of two primary hormones, *estrogen* and *progesterone,* in the ovaries. Both hormones work to change a girl into a woman physically and emotionally. They stimulate what we consider naturally feminine qualities: gentleness, passivity, and nurturance.

Estrogen causes growth of the breasts, widening of the hips, and maturation of the genitals, including the clitoris and the labia (which will be discussed later). In addition, a special lining called the *endometrium* in the girl's uterus begins to form in preparation for child bearing.

One of the primary signs of puberty in a girl, however, is the onset of menstruation, which we have discussed in the previous chapter. Puberty brings sexual maturity to both boys and girls. It does not, however, bring emotional maturity. That is a lifelong process.

EMOTIONAL INSTABILITY

As our children begin to mature sexually and change physically, they also experience emotional traumas. In most children, passage into adolescence is characterized by tremendous highs and lows of emotion. They become acutely aware of peer pressures in school, where they feel tremendous pressure to conform to what is considered "hip" or "cool" among their classmates. These worldly values usually conflict with the Christian values they have been taught at home.

Teenagers gradually begin to think independently of their parents and choose to make up their own mind about the world, their values, and religious convictions. It is essential that teenagers be active in a vital church youth group during this time so that some of the strongest influences from outside do not conflict with the family's. Fortunately, this can be a time when they are often open to spiritual challenges from God about what to do with their lives. A good church can help the whole family guide an adolescent over the rough spots of growing up.

An adolescent's mental processes fluctuate from child-like to adult thinking. He often feels confused about himself, his goals, his reason for living, and his relationships. He fights to be treated as an adult, but there is still that part of him that needs the comfort and security he knew as a child. In many ways, he wants the benefits of adulthood but not its responsibilities.

As he changes physically, an adolescent typically becomes uncomfortable with his looks. With his hormones in a state of flux, he will begin to notice oily skin, blackheads, or acne on his face. He may not like the shape of his nose. He may be embarrassed by his sudden growth spurt that sends him towering above everyone else in the classroom. Sudden growth often leaves a teen clumsy and uncoordinated for a time, which compounds his problems. Or he may feel like a dwarf because everyone else has grown three inches during the year and he's still four-eleven. What is worse, the girl he wanted to be friends with is suddenly six inches taller than he. So he worries about his attractiveness to girls.

I doubt that anything is more traumatic for a preadolescent boy or girl than the junior high school locker room. Early developers have the emotional edge over the late bloomers in the locker room, where everyone's physical attributes or lack thereof become painfully obvious. Those who have not yet entered puberty invariably compare their bodies with those who are physically more matured. The results can be disastrous. Depression and poor self-esteem are natural consequences when children unwisely compare their bodies with others in the locker room.

Children troubled by their lack of development should be reassured that their individual hormonal clocks are not broken—they are merely slower than others. Although a child who develops early has a slight advantage over a late bloomer, the former can also suffer self-esteem problems if he grows too tall or too wide.

As parents we need to understand the confusion, peer pressure, hormonal imbalances, and self-esteem problems that face our preadolescent children. They need extra amounts of loving patience from us. All children need love, but our love is going to be severely tested during their adolescence. We should be prepared for this.

Communicating with our children in an open, responsive way is one of the keys to getting through this traumatic time. We have to let our preadolescents know that they can come to us at any time and discuss any subject on their minds. They need to know that we are going to love them, pray for them, and comfort them during their journey from childhood to adulthood.

Preadolescents also need to know that we are going to continue to set guidelines for their behavior. These guidelines include such concerns as what kinds of friends they have, how they entertain themselves, and what their spiritual obligations are. Remember that we are still under the mandate from God to bring up our child in "the nurture and admonition of the Lord." Although we want a close relationship with our children, it is not advisable to enter into a "buddy" relationship with them. We are not to relinquish our God-given authority over them as long as they remain under our roof. Our real test will come when we are forced to demonstrate our love for them by being willing to endure their flak after we have had to say "no" to something.

SEXUAL MATURITY

Before our children enter adolescence, they should have a good understanding of their reproductive organs and how they are supposed to function. The following description builds on the information provided in previous chapters. The diagrams in chapters 3 and 4 will be helpful.

The Male Reproductive System

The male reproductive system includes the penis, glans penis, scrotum, sperm, Cowper's gland, urethra, testicles, vas deferens, ampulla, seminal vesicles, epididymis, and the prostate gland.

*The **penis** is, of course, a dual-purpose organ, used not only for sexual reproduction but also for eliminating waste liquids from the bladder. The tube inside the penis is called the **urethra**. The sperm cells pass through the penis into the woman's vagina during sexual intercourse. The inside of the penis is somewhat like a sponge, honeycombed with an* intricate network of tiny blood vessels. When a man is sexually aroused, these vessels fill with blood and the penis enlarges and becomes stiff. Valves within the blood vessels close, preventing the blood from leaving. This enlarged, stiff state is called an **erection.** An erection can occur at almost any time once a boy has entered puberty; it can occur not only from sexual arousal but also from nonstimulating conditions as simple as wearing tight-fitting clothing.

The head of the penis, called the **glans penis,** is one of the most sensitive areas of the body. This particular "erogenous zone" comprises densely packed nerves and is the main source of physical pleasure for a man in sexual intercourse.

The **scrotum** is the small bag of skin that contains the testicles. Also called **testes,** the **testicles** are oval glands about the size and shape of large nuts. Inside each testicle is a long tube about one-thousandth of an inch in diameter and about a thousand feet long. One testicle can produce as many as 500 million sperm cells each day. For sperm to be healthy, they must be manufactured in an environment about four degrees cooler than the normal human body temperature. That is why the testicles hang outside the body. In cold weather the muscles of the scrotum draw the testicles closer to the body to maintain the proper temperature within the scrotum. The scrotum itself has a unique design; the left part of the scrotum is slightly lower than the right one. This is to prevent the testicles from rubbing together when a man walks.

The testicles manufacture sperm cells every day. As the testicles fill up, the sperm pass into a tube known as the **epididymis,** inside the scrotal sac, where they mature. This is like an incubator or storage area.

As more and more sperm are produced, the mature sperm cells are transferred from the epididymis into a tube called the **vas deferens.** (In Latin, vas means "vessel" and deferens means "carry.") . From this tube they are deposited in another storage area called the **ampulla chamber.** The sperm eventually leave the ampulla chamber and enter the seminal vesicles, two organs that manufacture seminal fluid, or semen.

The male reproductive system includes two other important glands: the **prostate** and **Cowper's gland.** The prostate lies between the bladder and the base of the penis. It produces seminal fluid and contains nerves that control penile erections. It also contracts to help ejaculate sperm from the penis. Cowper's gland is the first gland to function when a man becomes sexually aroused. It sends a few drops of slippery fluid into the urethra, thus preparing it for the safe passage of sperm by neutralizing the acids of the urine that would otherwise kill the sperm. A valve at the top of the urethra opens to let urine out, but automatically shuts when sperm cells are on the way.

A sperm cell is an amazing creation. Under a microscope it looks like a tadpole. It has three parts. The head contains the chromosomes that will help determine the characteristics of the child should an egg be fertilized during intercourse. The neck contains the energy source to propel the sperm. The tail provides the sperm with the ability to travel through the vagina and into the Fallopian tube to meet the egg.

The egg is surrounded by several layers of protective material that the sperm must penetrate in order for conception to occur. The sperm has chemicals called enzymes that dissolve the layers around the egg and permit a sperm cell to burrow its way inside. The layers are so tough, it takes literally millions of these sperm to surround the egg and weaken the layers enough for a sperm to enter and fertilize an egg.

Intercourse doesn't always result in conception. Moreover, when it does, there are normally only one sperm cell and one egg involved. In rare instances, however, the fertilized egg divides in such a way that two babies begin to grow; this is how identical twins form. These babies will look exactly alike because they have the same combination of genes. At other times, two eggs are fertilized by different sperm at the same time, and this is how fraternal twins are conceived. Fraternal twins do not look alike, because they have a different combination of genes.

The Female Reproductive System

The female reproductive system has two parts, the external genitalia and the internal reproductive organs. The **vulva**, the external sexual organ that leads to the vagina, comprises several organs. The two large, fleshy folds of skin that cover the genitals are called the **labia majora**. (In Latin, labia means "lips" and majora means "large.") Located just inside the labia majora are two smaller folds of skin, the **labia minora**. Right at the top of the labia minora is a tiny, pea-shaped organ called the **clitoris**. The clitoris is located near the **urethra**, the opening where waste liquid is eliminated.

The clitoris is equivalent to a man's penis except that it is much smaller. Like a penis, it has a **glans** at the top and a small shaft. As in a man, the glans is densely filled with nerve endings; this makes it a woman's most sensitive sexual organ. Unlike the penis, however, the clitoris has no opening at the end and plays no part in reproduction itself.

The **hymen**, deriving its name from the mythical Greek god of marriage, is a membrane at the back part of the outside opening of the vagina. This membrane partly covers the vaginal entrance.

A woman's internal sexual organs include the vagina, ovaries, Fallopian tubes, uterus, and cervix. The **vagina** is the birth canal through which the baby passes from the uterus to the outside of the mother's body. (Vagina is Latin for "sheath" or "scabbard.") The vagina is from three to five inches long. Its walls contain many tiny glands that secrete a cleansing liquid to keep the area free from germs.

The **uterus**, which is a Latin word meaning "womb" or "belly," is the size and shape of a pear, about four inches long. This is where the baby will grow for nine months until he is ready to be born. Two **Fallopian tubes** are attached to the top of the uterus. These tubes lead toward the **ovaries**, where unfertilized eggs are stored. Although it is not directly connected to the ovary, a Fallopian tube catches the egg when it is released from the ovary.

An egg is normally in the Fallopian tube when fertilization takes place. It then continues its journey into the uterus, propelled through the Fallopian tube by tiny hairs called **cilia**. If the egg is not fertilized, it dissolves and comes out of the woman's body during the **menstrual period**. If the egg is fertilized, it will attach itself to the uterine wall in a few days for the gestation process.

At the lower end of the uterus is the **cervix**, which is Latin for "neck." This connects the uterus to the vagina. The opening of the cervix is usually only about the diameter of a pencil lead, but it expands greatly when the baby is ready to be born.

NOCTURNAL EMISSIONS

Adolescent sex drives are strong. They are healthy drives as long as they are kept under control and channeled in the right directions. It is important that our children understand that even a powerful sexual drive is normal and controllable. First Corinthians 10:13 informs us that we need not be overpowered sexually to violate the laws and principles of God. Moreover, medical experts tell us that no physical damage results when sexual tension is not released. We should communicate this to our preadolescents and inform them as well of the unique release mechanism for boys known as nocturnal emission.

If a boy is not properly prepared for it, a *nocturnal emission,* or "wet dream," can be a disturbing experience. Awakening in the middle of the night to find his sheets wet from semen is unsettling and often produces feelings of guilt or shame. These feelings can be alleviated if a boy is given a simple explanation of what is happening. In the male reproductive system, God created a unique release mechanism for unused sperm cells, which are produced by the thousands every day.

Eventually there are so many sperm cells that the storage places (the epididymis, seminal vesicles, and prostate gland) are full. What happens then is a little like what happens when a pot of water boils over on the stove; the water bubbles up and over the edge of the pot. When the male reproductive system is filled to overflowing with sperm cells, the penis becomes particularly sensitive to any external stimulation—even something as simple as rubbing against bedsheets at night. A little stimulation is enough to cause the penis to expel some of the sperm to relieve the pressure on the storage places. In many cases, a full bladder pressing against the seminal vesicle will result in ejaculation at night.

Often a nocturnal emission is accompanied by a sexually oriented dream. Ejaculation is a sexual experience, so it's not unusual that a sexually stimulating dream would accompany it. Dreams are subconscious, and a boy need not feel guilt or shame when this experience occurs, for God knows he has no control over his brain while sleeping.

The "wet dream" is God's method of releasing the buildup of sperm cells and sexual energy in an adolescent boy or in a man. It is easier for a boy to learn about this from his father, but frequently a mother discovers the signs of a wet dream when changing her son's sheets. We should reassure our sons that this is all very normal and they need not feel embarrassed.

By keeping a casual, matter-of-fact attitude we can convey positive feelings about wet dreams to our sons. They should come to see them as a gift from God for helping the body to take care of itself.

MASTURBATION

Masturbation is a common practice among teens, particularly boys. Therefore it seems wise to include a discussion of it in this chapter. The following discussion of masturbation comes from my book *The Act of Marriage:*

"Is It Wrong for a Christian to Masturbate?

"There is probably no more controversial question in the field of sex than this. A few years ago every Christian would have given an unqualified yes, but that was before the sexual revolution and before doctors declared that the practice is not harmful to health. No longer can a father honestly warn his son that it will cause 'brain damage, weakness, baldness, blindness, epilepsy, or insanity.' Some still refer to it as 'self-abuse' and 'sinful behavior'; others advocate it as a necessary relief to the single man and a help for the married man whose wife is pregnant or whose business forces him to be away from home for long periods of time.

"To show the influence of humanism on people's decisions, we found it interesting that in our survey of twenty-five Christian doctors, 72 percent approved masturbation and 28 percent felt it is wrong. By contrast, among pastors (whose graduate-school training was in seminary and undergraduate education often in a Christian college) only 13 percent approved self-manipulation and 83 percent considered it wrong. In most cases, ministers are not uninformed on the subject; they probably have to cope with it in the counseling room more than doctors. Certainly they deal with it among single men through their camp and youth programs.

"Among those who took our survey, 52 percent of the men and 84 percent of women declared they had never or seldom practiced masturbation; 17 percent of men and 4 percent of women indicated they had practiced masturbation frequently or regularly. Many of these stated specifically they no longer did so since becoming a Christian.

"Unfortunately the Bible is silent on this subject; therefore it is dangerous to be dogmatic. Although we are sympathetic with those who would remove the time-honored taboos against the practice, we would like to suggest the following reasons why we do not feel it is an acceptable practice for Christians:

"1. Fantasizing and lustful thinking are usually involved in masturbation, and the Bible clearly condemns such thoughts (Matt. 5:28).

"2. Sexual expression was designed by God to be performed jointly by two people of the opposite sex, resulting in a necessary and healthy dependence on each other for the experience. Masturbation frustrates that designed dependence.

"3. Guilt is a universal aftermath of masturbation unless one has been brainwashed by the humanistic philosophy that does not believe in a God-given conscience or, in many cases, right and wrong. Such guilt interferes with spiritual growth and produces defeat in single young people particularly. To them it is usually a self-discipline hurdle they must scale in order to grow in Christ and walk in the Spirit.

"4. It violates 1 Corinthians 7:9: 'For it is better to marry than to burn.' If a young man practices masturbation, it tends to nullify a necessary and important motivation for marriage. There are already enough social, educational, and financial demotivators on young men now; they don't need this one.

"5. It creates a habit before marriage that can easily be resorted to afterward as a cop-out when a husband and wife have sexual or other conflicts that make coitus difficult.

"6. It defrauds a wife (1 Cor. 7:3–5). No married man should relieve his mounting, God-given desire for his wife except through coitus. She will feel unloved and insecure, and many little problems will unnecessarily be magnified by this artificial draining of his sex drive. This becomes increasingly true as a couple reach middle age."[1]

There are many differences of opinion on this subject among Christian pastors, doctors, psychologists, and psychiatrists. In his book *Sexual Understanding Before Marriage,*

Herbert J. Miles, a sociologist and former pastor, states that a young man should depend upon nocturnal emissions to release his pent-up sexual energy. He also believes, however, that a "limited and temporary" program of masturbation is appropriate for late adolescents. Miles believes that it is permissible as long as the masturbation is done for purposes of self-control and is not based on lustful thoughts. (Personally I question whether it can be done without such thoughts, particularly for adults.)

Psychologist James Dobson writes in his book, *Preparing for Adolescence:*

> Unfortunately, I can't speak directly for God on this subject, since His Holy Word, the Bible, is silent at this point. I will tell you what I *believe*, although I certainly do not want to contradict what your parents or your pastor believe. It is my *opinion* that masturbation is not much of an issue with God. It's a normal part of adolescence which involves no one else. It does not cause disease, it does not produce babies, and Jesus did not mention it in the Bible. I'm not telling you to masturbate, and I hope you won't feel the need for it. But if you do, it is my opinion that you should not struggle with guilt over it.[2]

SEXUAL ROLES AND SEX DEVIATIONS

Ever since the feminist and homosexual movements began gaining notoriety in the news media, there has been a trend in our society toward the "unisex" look. The unisex style of dress and behavior began to become popular during the 1960s among the "flower children" and has continued to this day. Boy George and other rock stars are promoting it by openly affirming transvestism.

Adolescents are going through enough trauma without also suffering from this sex-role confusion intentionally fostered by Boy George and his ilk. Much sex-role differentiation is learned behavior. Boys should look to men as role models of what constitutes proper masculine behavior; girls should depend on women to show them what is proper feminine behavior.

Teenagers must understand that there is a basic, God-created difference between males and females. The difference is not just physical; it extends even to the construction of the brain. Thinking patterns, emotions, and attitudes are all different. Men think more logically than women, but women have an intuition that often proves more accurate than "logic." Men are more "work oriented"; women are more oriented toward the "home" and "people."

The sex hormones produced in males and females give them their masculine or feminine characteristics. Estrogen and progesterone in women produce qualities such as gentleness, nurturing, and passivity. In men, the hormone testosterone gives them their attributes of aggressiveness, dominance, ambition, and sexual initiative.

Dr. W. Peter Blitchington points out in his book on sex roles that scientific studies have determined that an excessive amount of testosterone can actually cause a female's brain to be masculinized. A girl whose brain has been dosed with testosterone in the womb will have aggressive characteristics. Likewise, a boy who has not received the proper amount of testosterone will have a feminized brain and will exhibit feminine characteristics. Blitchington points out that if testosterone is blocked from the central nervous system during the seventh week of development of a fetus, a male will tend to be passive and effeminate.

God created males and females with complementary sex characteristics so that when they were joined together in marriage, these characteristics would make a "whole" or complete sexual unit. God designed men and women with opposing characteristics so they would need each other's strengths and could help each other overcome their weaknesses.

Dr. Blitchington observes, "By design, all of God's creation is constructed to avoid self-sufficiency. Everything about our earth and its inhabitants is designed to promote harmony, interdependence, and unselfishness."[3]

Our adolescents should understand that their particular attitudes and feelings are God-given. It is God's will that a young man be aggressive in his work. It is God's will that a young woman have a desire to bear children. God places these desires and drives in males and females for mutual pleasure and the survival of the race. However, people's temperaments will also influence the expression of these innate desires to some extent.

In this age of sexual confusion, it is important for our children to have positive role models to reinforce the God-given sexual attributes present in them. A boy needs to see his father as someone who is strong and decisive, who effectively leads his family, but who is also a loving and caring person. A boy needs to be trained in the skills he will need if he is to be a competent provider of his own family someday. Most important in a boy's life is proper spiritual training; he must be taught about his responsibility as the head of a family. The best way to teach this is through example and a consistent Christian life. A girl also needs a role model to learn from. Her mother can provide that guidance by teaching her about the home and training her for motherhood.

What I am describing is preparation for our children to have traditional families someday. In human history there has never been a substitute for the traditional family (comprising a father, mother, and children living in a common area). Anthropologists who have studied both primitive and civilized societies have found the traditional family to be a consistent pattern throughout recorded history. I point out in my book *The Battle for the Family,* "Anthropologist George P. Murdock, who analyzed some five hundred cultures, found only one society that lacked the basic family unit as we know it, and it is extinct!"[4] That extinct society is the Nayars of southern India. While their culture existed, a man would visit a woman's tent at night, impregnate her, and leave. The mother and her female relatives would rear the child. Little wonder this tribe is now extinct! God's formula for the family is the only one that works. It is the most effective way of rearing children and preparing them for adulthood.

Within the traditional family we find that males and females have different but complementary roles. The male has traditionally been the hunter or provider; the female has prepared the food and cared for the children. This pattern has provided stability to the culture, whether primitive or civilized.

Whenever this pattern has been distorted or corrupted, the society has inevitably declined. In *Our Dance Has Turned to Death,* Carl Wilson discusses the dangers of sex-role confusion and notes that there are common characteristics of civilizations in decline.

The pattern in ancient Greece, in the Roman Republic and in America is the same:

1. Men ceased to lead their families in worship. Spiritual and moral development became secondary. Their view of God became more naturalistic, mathematical, and mechanical.

2. Men selfishly neglected the care of their wives and children to pursue material wealth, political and military power, and cultural development. Material values began to dominate thought, and the man began to exalt his own role as an individual.

3. Men, being preoccupied with business or war, either neglected their wives sexually or became involved with lower-class women or with homosexuality, and a double standard of morality developed.

4. The role of women at home and with children lost value and status. Women, being neglected and their roles devalued, revolted to gain access to material wealth and also freedom for sex outside of marriage. Women began to minimize having sex relations to conceive children, and the emphasis became sex for pleasure. Laws regulating marriage made divorce easy.

5. Husbands and wives competed against each other for money, home leadership, and the affection of their children, resulting in hostility and frustration and possible homosexuality in the children. Many marriages ended in separation and

divorce. Many children were unwanted, aborted, abandoned, molested, and undisciplined. The more undisciplined children became, the more social pressure there was not to have children. The breakdown of the home produced anarchy.

6. Selfish individualism grew and was carried over into society, fragmenting it into smaller and smaller group loyalties. The nation was thus weakened by internal conflict. The decrease in the birthrate produced an older population that had less ability to defend itself and less will to do so, making the nation more vulnerable to its enemies.

7. As unbelief in God became more complete and parental authority diminished, ethical and moral principles disappeared, affecting the economy and government. Thus, by internal weakness and fragmentation the societies came apart. There was no way to save them except by a dictator who arose from within or invaded from without.[5]

The confusion of sex roles in our society is leading to role reversal and the destruction of God's design for men, women, and children. Men are being feminized and women are becoming masculinized in their attitudes and actions. Our whole civilization will be seriously undermined if we continue to allow our culture to be debased by the philosophies of feminism and the militancy of the homosexual movement.

For additional reading on sexual roles in boys and girls, I recommend George A. Rekers' book, *Shaping Your Child's Sexual Identity*,* and W. Peter Blitchington's book, *Sex Roles and the Christian Family.*

HOMOSEXUALITY

In recent years we have heard a great deal about homosexuals and their lifestyle. They are not a new phenomenon; they have been with us at least since the days of Lot (Genesis 17). However, they seem to be increasing in number and have

---

*Grand Rapids: Baker Book House, 1982.

"come out of their closets" and are demanding the right to take positions as teachers in our public schools. Most Christians oppose this because they do not wish to give them a captive audience of impressionable young minds on which to extol their lifestyle.

Although they would like us to believe they are "born homosexual," the truth is, no scientific evidence has come to light that suggests that conclusion. Instead, it is usually a combination of several things that makes a person a homosexual.

As I noted in my book *What Everyone Should Know About Homosexuality,* there are eight major factors that may predispose a young man or woman to turn to homosexual behavior.

1. *Temperament.* I have found that most homosexuals reflect a high degree of melancholy temperament. They are usually sensitive, artistic, gifted, introverted perfectionists who were very impressionable in their youth. Most were rejected by one parent or sibling, and by the time they reach adulthood are extremely angry.

2. *Inadequate parental relationships.* One professor of psychiatry notes, "Current research indicates that the family most likely to produce a homosexual comprises a very intimate, possessive and dominating mother and a detached, hostile father. Many mothers of lesbians tend to be hostile and competitive with their daughters. The fathers of female homosexuals seldom appear to play a dominant role in the family and have considerable difficulty being openly affectionate with their daughters."[6]

3. *Permissive childhood training.* In studying the case histories of numerous homosexuals, it became obvious to me that they were either pampered or rejected as children. They have such a lack of discipline in their lives that it is easy for them to fall into a homosexual lifestyle.

4. *Insecurity about sexual identity.* Many parents have

unknowingly damaged their children by refusing to accept them for what they are. Often when a father has a daughter but wanted a son, he will treat her like a boy. This kind of rejection from parents can make children reject their own sex and seek to imitate the opposite sex. I wrote in *What Everyone Should Know About Homosexuality,* "It is important for girls to accept their femininity and enjoy being women, while boys should be trained to esteem their manhood. Learning to love and accept yourself is fundamental to learning to love someone else."[7]

5. *Childhood sexual trauma.* Sexual exploitation or molestation damages children and may lead them into a homosexual or promiscuous lifestyle. Many boys are led into homosexuality by older boys or men who have befriended them for sexual reasons before puberty begins. Consequently they are guided in the wrong direction and develop the habit of homosexuality. In all likelihood, if they had been left alone, they would naturally have grown up heterosexual. Unfortunately, each experience fosters habits, guilt patterns, and thought processes that may lead to homosexual practices.

6. *Early interest in sex.* Studies of homosexual males show that many entered puberty earlier than other boys and began masturbating earlier. This early fascination with sex can be particularly damaging when there is no natural outlet for sexual energy. Since most of a boy's friends in preadolescence are other boys, early puberty and its concomitant fascination with sex may lead to homosexual experimentation.

7. *Youthful masturbation and sexual fantasizing.* Most of the homosexuals I know indulged in masturbation early and frequently. This seems to be a crucial step in adopting a homosexual lifestyle. As frequent masturbators, they learn to associate their genitals with sexual pleasure. This association can overcome heterosexual leanings and destroy a natural

attraction toward females. Masturbation and fantasizing can divert a child from normal sexual desires and serve as a catalyst that will provide him with a mental attitude favorable to homosexuality.

8. *Childhood associates and peer pressure.* Many young boys possessing feminine characteristics have been unmercifully teased as children. This teasing or rejection can result in self-hatred. If a boy has been rejected by his friends or worse still, by his father, he may accentuate his feminine characteristics and drift toward homosexuality. Our children's friends may also be a bad influence on them by introducing them to sexual experimentation. Molestation from caregivers, such as baby sitters or workers in day-care centers, can also be harmful.

These eight conditions are some of the factors that may lead children into a homosexual lifestyle. Homosexuality is not a biological reality; it is a learned behavior. It is the result of a process that begins with a combination of these eight factors, is reinforced by an initial homosexual experience, and becomes a habit because of increasingly pleasurable thoughts and feelings and experiences with members of the same sex. The more our children expose themselves to homosexual thoughts, the more likely they are to be drawn into that lifestyle.

Once involved in homosexuality, a person finds the habit difficult to break. The more a person fantasizes frequently about members of his own sex, the easier it becomes to try to fulfill the fantasies. With repeated episodes of homosexual behavior, the boy's sexual orientation is gradually steered away from heterosexuality. If homosexual thought patterns become entrenched in a child's mind before he reaches puberty, his increased sex drive after puberty will intensify toward his own sex—not, as it should, toward the opposite sex.

How to Protect Children From Homosexuality

A child is best protected from homosexuality by being brought up in a decent Christian home where the father is the loving head of the home; where the mother is supportive of the father's role and where she has warm and affectionate relationships with her sons and daughters.

In his excellent study of homosexuality, *Growing Up Straight,* George Rekers writes, "A secure and normal sexual identity in a child is best fostered by a stable home where both father and mother provide affection, attention, and security for their children."[8] If children are growing up in a home where there is a single parent of the opposite sex, every effort should be made to provide a same-sex role model for them. For example, a boy could look to an uncle or grandfather as a role model. A girl could look to her big sister, aunt or another positive female as a model for her behavior.

The key to protecting our children from homosexuality is for us to study and obey the Scriptures and to live the Word of God in our own lives. By paying attention to our children, by loving them, communicating with them, and listening to them, we will most likely have success in raising sons and daughters who have no sex-role confusion or leanings toward homosexuality. I say "most likely," because no matter how good we are as parents, our children will eventually exercise their free wills and deliberately choose one lifestyle over another. If we are committed believers who have done everything in our power to bring up godly children and one goes astray, I don't think we can take the blame on ourselves. God gave each of us a free will either to accept or to reject His salvation. That same free will allows our children to reject everything we have ever taught them—regardless of how hard we have tried to help them live according to God's Word.

DOING OUR JOBS

It is becoming increasingly apparent that just teaching our children is not enough. We must protect them from the wrong influences at this tender age. It is a wise parent who knows where and with whom his eleven-to-thirteen-year-old is at all times—and to be "watchful," as the Scriptures teach. Remember, homosexuals that would misdirect your son or daughter don't wear badges saying, "I am a homosexual." Quite the opposite—they do everything they can to appear normal.

As parents we have the responsibility to convey our moral values and these truths about sexual matters to our preadolescents to prepare them for adulthood. Waiting for them to bring up the subject may prove fruitless. We need to initiate the discussion. How to do this is considered in the next chapter.

6

Teenagers

SURVEYS INDICATE that four out of five teenagers rarely talk to their parents about sex. Yet most indicate they would like to do so. One of the surveys asked, "Whom would you most like to talk to you about sex: teacher, counselor, minister, friends, parents? The majority responded, "My parents."

As a child grows into his teen years, both his interest in the subject of sex and the need to know increase dramatically. Because of the changing forces going on inside him, he thinks about sex more than ever and talks about it with his friends, who are as uninformed as he. Because of teenagers' adult physical capabilities and the enormous sexual pressures placed on them by our culture, it is imperative that parents talk to their children about sex at this age, particularly if they haven't discussed it together during the younger years.

Whose job is it to begin the discussion of sex? Most parents have the mistaken idea that "if my son wants to talk to me about sex, he will ask." Actually, he won't. As we have already been informed, sex is the most difficult subject in the world for parents and children to talk about, particularly when humor is omitted and values and responsibility are included. It becomes a sensitive issue, making both parties very self-conscious. If a parent who is waiting for his teenager to bring up the subject really understood the conflict going on in his youngster, he would force himself to open the conversational door. After all, he has a vested interest in whether or not his teen is prepared for this major facet of life. Moreover, if he had never talked to his child about the subject in order to develop a free and open spirit toward it, he may emote fear and a feeling of distaste that the youth picks up and mistakenly reads as "Dad (or Mother) wants to stay clear of this subject."

There is usually a certain amount of question in the mind of teenagers on this subject. He has developed feelings never experienced before and he sometimes has to fight off impure thoughts not wrestled with earlier in life. As one young person admitted, "I'm afraid my parents will think I'm doing the things I ask them about."

I have discovered a great amount of hostility toward parents from teenagers who are in trouble over sex (pregnancy, premarital sex, VD, etc.). While it is true that many get into trouble because they rebel against their parents, they may also feel resentful toward parents who never talked to them about sex, concluding that such discussions might have forestalled their mistakes. A survey that supports this indicated that while most young people prefer to learn about sex from their parents, four out of five who were in trouble did not want to talk to their parents about it.

The evidence is convincing that as difficult as it may be to introduce the subject, it is a parent's right and duty to do so. Even when our teens show embarrassment and temporary reluctance we must make sure to leave the door open. Sometimes a teen will reflect on the fact that he responded to an initial conversation badly and will be more receptive the next time. Leave your son or daughter with the impression that "anytime you want to talk, I am ready to do so. No subject is too small or too personal for you to discuss with me."

Probably the best way to initiate a conversation is to ask our teens the questions that are most likely to be on their minds. This should be done by the parent of the same sex when possible. Surveys indicate that the following questions reflect the major concerns of most young people depending on their ages.

FATHERS' QUESTIONS TO SONS

When introducing the subject of sex into a conversation with our teens we should try to be as casual as possible. Remember, we usually know in advance what we are going to talk about, but the teens are caught by surprise. We should look them in the eye and say something like this: "Jim, we haven't talked about sex for some time now. Would you mind if I asked you a question?" Usually the teen thinks, "Good grief, he's going to ask if I've had sex with a girl!" so he is relieved when we ask a much less threatening question. The day may come when we should ask that question, but it is hardly the one with which to open the conversational door.

We may also begin, "I'd like to have a talk with you about sex, Jim. It may be uncomfortable for both of us at first, but it's so important that I think we should discuss it anyway. You are approaching manhood, and you will find that the sexual forces and changes going on inside you will have a powerful effect on your whole life."

Question (early teens): Have you started to feel your sex drive increase lately? Let him respond. You might add, *Does it bother you?* Notice how unthreatening that question is. It assumes these are natural feelings and if he hasn't experienced them yet, he will. Never lecture or preach at him, but offer brief explanations of things you feel he is old enough to ask. At times you can identify with him by observing, *I remember when I was your age. I felt guilty when I had these feelings, and it wasn't until later that I found it was natural— all the guys had them.*

Perhaps you can add, *When I was your age, my dad and I enjoyed some great talks about sex that really helped me prepare for manhood. I hope we can have talks like that too.* If you can't say that, you can at least set the stage so he can make that remark to his son some day.

Question: Has it made it difficult for you to concentrate on your studies, your spiritual life or Bible reading?

Question: Do you think a lot about girls? You may wish to add, *Do you know what Jesus meant when He talked about lusting being as bad as adultery?* With this you might wish to read Matthew 5:27–28.

Question: Do you know what causes a man to have a sex drive? If he does not understand, it will be helpful to review the material in the preceding chapter. He needs to identify the sex drive as a gift of God, a natural drive that must be controlled.

Question: Have you had any wet dreams yet? Most boys awaken from a wet dream feeling guilty. They should understand that this is God's merciful gift of "overflow" when his body manufactures more sperm cells and semen than his system can handle. He should also be told that the dream does not cause the emission but is caused by the sexual overflow. If his body had not manufactured so much sexual fluid, he would not have experienced the dream. However, he does need to be counseled to avoid pornography or sexually lurid TV programs and movies, for they cause the dreams as well. For additional information on this important subject, see the section on "Wet Dreams" in the chapter "What All Parents Need to Know to Talk To Their Children About Sex."

Question: Have you had a problem with masturbation yet? This is probably one of the toughest questions for your son to answer. He needs your assurance that as a man you understand that almost all men have experienced masturbation. According to an old saying, "99 percent of all men have masturbated at one time or another, and the other 1 percent are liars." I did meet one young man who claimed he had never done it, and because of the dedicated minister he is today, I believe him. But he is rare indeed. This too is a subject you should study in the preceding chapter to be properly informed.

Question: Do you fully understand how babies are conceived? This provides an opportunity to determine how much he knows. Be sure to listen intently to his description, letting him describe what he knows. If you have done your work well in the lower grades, you will not have to teach much here. It is important, however, that you are not critical of what he doesn't know. Tell him, *That's good, Jim. There are just a couple of things I'd like to add.* Then provide the necessary additions.

Question: How old does a girl have to be before she can get pregnant? You may be surprised by his answer. Explain that she becomes fertile after she has started to menstruate.

Question: How many teens your age do you think are sexually active? The statistics on this are alarming. Surveys are so diverse that they prove nothing except that young people are more active today than at any time in American history. Some estimates go as high as 73 percent for boys and 58 percent for girls. It is assumed that 50 percent are sexually active before graduation from high school. Even Christian young people are sexually more active than they were ten years ago. Most parents, ministers, and Christian school officials would be amazed at the sexual activity of youth coming from Christian homes. Do not assume that your son "wouldn't do it." It is important for both of you to start talking early so that he will know that some day you will look him in the eye and ask if he has ever had intercourse with a girl. That prospect alone might cool him down some night when his passions have all but run away with him.

Question: Do you know any promiscuous girls? You don't need any names. Indeed it is important to assure your son that you will keep his confidence. Don't even tell your wife what he shares privately unless you get his permission.

Question: Would you date a promiscuous girl?

Question: Do you know any girls who have become pregnant in high school?

Question: What do you know about venereal disease? Your son should know something about syphilis, gonorrhea, and herpes and should understand that the last is incurable and is reaching epidemic proportions. The last chapter of this book has more information.

Question: What do you know about AIDS? This fearful strain of VD is now breaking out of the homosexual community and has become a real danger to prostitutes and their customers, blood receivers, and in some cases the medical profession.

Questions: Do you have any homosexual friends? or *Do you know any boys who are gay?* On the one hand, you do not want to implant hatred for homosexuals in the heart of your son. On the other hand, you don't want him to make them his dearest friends. Gays are not usually difficult to spot even if they have not come out of the closet. They tend to be hostile people and will have a detrimental influence on your son. Unless they are repentant homosexuals seeking God's grace and power to overcome their homosexuality, you should not permit your son to run around with them. Remember the apostle Paul's words, "Evil companions corrupt good morals."

Additional Questions You May Ask Your Son

Question: What do you think about oral sex? This question should be asked of your son at about age sixteen or seventeen if he is dating a girl regularly. It should not be asked by itself and should be introduced gently. But you should inquire, because oral sex is probably the most common form of birth control used today by teens before marriage.

Other potential questions:

- *Did God give us sex only for making babies?*
- *Do you know why girls menstruate?*
- *Are you aware of the emotional pressure a girl feels when she menstruates?*
- *How should a boy treat a girl if he knows she is having her period?*
- *Does a young man need premarital sex experience in order to be a good love partner when he gets married?*
- *What do you know about abortion?*
- *What is your honest feeling about abortion for an unwed teenage girl?*
- *What do you think is the boy's responsibility in the matter of abortion?*
- *Do you know what the Bible teaches about premarital sex?*
- *What passages come to mind?*
- *Is there a difference between adultery and fornication?*
- *How far can a couple go?*

Reasons You Can Give Your Son for Waiting to Have Sex

In an age when teens are subjected to enormous pressures to experiment with sex and treat it casually, a boy needs some *reasons* why he should delay that activity until marriage. He may be in a typical public school, where some sex educators openly teach or infer that teens "ought to practice their sexuality" or "have the right to control their own bodies" or "make their own choices." Parents are left with the responsibility of helping their teens pick up the pieces of their shattered lives.

A teenager can hardly watch television without viewing a

passionate show of affection that concludes in sexual relations, or infers it. TV studies reveal that explicit sex scenes occur 2.7 times an hour during prime time; more than three-quarters of these episodes are between unmarried people or homosexuals. That totals 13.5 times an evening or 67.5 times a week. Whose moral values are under attack? Yours. And your son's. With this and the many other sexually stimulating pressures of our society, not the least of which may be the pretty girlfriend he dates, he needs your help. She may be as innocent as he, but to remain that way, they both need to be armed at this time with logical reasons for not engaging in life's most exciting experience.

Many of their friends may already be promiscuous, and some may be pressuring them to conform to the new-age morality which is really the old immorality. Your son needs to hear *why* he shouldn't engage in premarital sex from *you.* Here are some suggestions.

1. *Your body belongs to God, not to you.* "Do you now know that your bodies are members of Christ himself? Shall I then take the members of Christ and unite them with a prostitute? Never! Do you not know that he who unites himself with a prostitute is one with her in body? For it is said, 'The two will become one flesh.' But he who unites himself with the Lord is one with him in spirit. Flee from sexual immorality. All other sins a man commits are outside his body, but he who sins sexually sins against his own body. Do you not know that your body is a temple of the Holy Spirit, who is in you, whom you have received from God? You are not your own; you were bought at a price. Therefore honor God with your body" (1 Corinthians 6:15–20).

Every teenager needs to understand that intercourse *except* between married partners is a sin against his body, which (if he is a Christian) is the temple of God. He defiles not only himself, but God's temple.

2. *Adultery is a sin, expressly forbidden by God seven times in Scripture.* "Thou shalt not commit adultery" (Exo-

dus 20:14. See also Deuteronomy 5:18; Matthew 5:27; 19:18; Luke 8:20; Romans 13:9; James 2:11).

3. *You are to be the spiritual leader in any close relationship you may have.* It is impossible to lead a girl spiritually if you have illicit sex with her. You have a responsibility toward God, your parents, her parents, the girl herself, and even her future husband to help her spiritually while you are going together. Dating can be an exciting time even without sexual activity. It supplies a vital need in the maturity process of every young person. Don't waste those months or years in adult behavior. You will cheat not only the future, but also the present.

4. *Your personal spiritual life depends on holiness of thought and practice.* To be the man God wants you to become, you must give some time in your life to spiritual maturity through Bible study, witnessing, and prayer. The adolescent years form a special period of development mentally, vocationally, socially, and spiritually. If your social life involves premarital sex, you will not develop spiritually at this very crucial period in your life.

5. *Premarital sex clouds your judgment at what could be the most important time in your life.* There are five major decisions you will probably make between the ages of eighteen and twenty-four that will affect the rest of your life. Engaging in premarital sex keeps you from making these decisions clearly and with God's blessing.

    a. Where will you go after high school? This may include college or training in a trade. Those who have gone to college admit that this has had a profound effect on their friends, choice of vocation, and future associations.

    b. What will be your vocation?

    c. Whom will you marry?

    d. Where will you work and live?

    e. Where will you go to church?

These questions will very likely chart the course of your life for the next fifty years. This is the time for clear-headed, Spirit-filled thinking. It is not the time to fall prey to an obsession with sex.

6. *Premarital sex could cause you to be faced with the responsibility of fathering an illegitimate child.* God has given you the gift of procreative life. Do you want a child whom you have fathered raised by someone else? Or do you wish to marry a girl before you can adequately support her and your child? What future is there for an illegitimate child compared with the happy home you have been raised in?

7. *Do you want the responsibility for ruining a girl's life?* Nothing can damage a young woman's life like an unplanned, unwanted pregnancy. This is a heavy weight to carry on your conscience. No amount of immediate excitement and pleasure can compensate for years of grief that such an act would cause so many people (the two of you, the child, and the grandparents).

8. *Do you want the responsibility of teaching a young girl to be promiscuous?* Premarital sex is usually initiated by two young people who love each other very much. They justify it by insisting that they would never give themselves to anyone else and that intimacy is permissible between two people in love. However, when they start having sex at age sixteen or eighteen, they will probably fall out of love but thereafter face an appetite for sex that makes it easier for them to be intimate with others.

Although it may seem unthinkable now, history shows that many prostitutes and promiscuous women gave their virtue to a man they loved during their teen years. You should never do on a date what you would not want another young man to do with your future wife.

9. *Treat every girl the way you wish other boys to treat your sister.* Dating is a sacred trust. You bear responsibility for another man's most treasured possession. Grant her the respect and decency that accompanies such trust.

10. *You must learn self-control and self-discipline.* Everyone knows that sex is exciting and pleasurable, but the foremost human trait every person needs in life is self-discipline. Denying yourself the opportunity of sex before marriage will never hurt you, but it will build character into your life and teach you that passions and desires can be controlled. Self-discipline in this matter will enable you to gain it in others. It takes a better man to say no than to say yes.

11. *You need to save your sexual expression for your one true love.* Nice girls, particularly Christian girls, sooner or later almost always ask their mate, "Have you ever had sex with another woman?" Will you be able to look her straight in the eye and reply with a clear conscience, "No"? If you can, her respect for you will soar, for she will realize that you are someone special. It is estimated that only 20 percent of the males in the United States enter marriage without sexual experience.

One advantage of your obvious self-control prior to marriage is that she can trust you more after marriage. If a man restrains himself from premarital sex, it is very likely he will resist the temptation to extramarital sex.

If we fathers study these questions and discussions, we will be armed to prepare our sons as few young men are prepared. The ensuing discussions will build a vital relationship between the father and son that will last a lifetime.

MOTHERS' QUESTIONS TO DAUGHTERS

Mother and daughters often have an easier time than fathers and sons in communicating about sex. Unless their temperaments are seriously in conflict, a daughter often looks to her mother for advice if she feels that her parents enjoy a positive relationship and if mother is not too critical and judgmental.

Nothing stifles communication between teens and parents like grating adult criticism. Teens are fond of shocking their parents with off-the-wall ideas they have borrowed from their peers. If parents respond by condemnation or harsh criticism of their friends, future communication sessions will be jeopardized. At times silence is a golden key to communication. By silence we are not giving assent to our children's latest "pipe dream," but we *are* letting the sound of their voices filter down into their base of reasoning in the light of our presence. That might be the time to ask, "How do you feel about that?" or "What do you think about that?" These two questions are normally asked only by parents who communicate with their teens. Parents should realize that these questions are excellent ways to help an emotionally bottled-up teen express himself. If we develop the habit of asking these two questions and listening without interruption, we will find the gates of communication opening wide and our daughters enjoying our openness and receptivity. Listening, not giving advice, is the essential ingredient of mother-daughter relationships.

We should be sure to develop one other quality in our promotion of dialogue: Try to be shockproof. Teens offer many pronouncements with a minimum of thought and express feelings that are temporary. Some simply love to shock their parents. Try responding, "Is that what you *really* think?" If we become shockproof, few barriers will be raised between us and our daughters, and they will feel they can share anything with us—as long as they can trust us. Like any good counselor, we must grant our "clients" the counseling privilege: never betray a confidence.

Some of the questions that fathers ask their sons are appropriate for mothers to use with slight modifications. You may wish to make your own adaptations of these. The weight of the questions will depend on the age level of the girl.

Questions About Menstruation

Girls and their mothers tend to talk more easily than boys and fathers because the onset of menstruation requires discussion and explanation. It is rare that a girl, no matter how close she is to her father, would go to him for counseling on this matter. It is more natural for a girl to confide in her mother. The first painful cramps usually cause her to seek parental help. I assume that you as a mother have prepared your daughter for this event. If not, use her first female cramps as a signal that you are behind and need to catch up. Apart from menstruation, a girl's development of breasts and pubic hair will necessitate frank mother-daughter talks around ages twelve to fourteen. Again, it is the mother's duty to open the conversational door, not the daughter's. By raising questions, you can attract her interest and make it easier for her to ask about things that are troubling her.

Question: One of the subjects we should discuss is menstruation. Would you like to talk about it now? This could be a tactful opening to an eleven-to-thirteen-year-old. You may want to refresh your knowledge on the subject by reading chapter 5 and then discuss with her the cause, process, and results. Be sure to include her emotional reactions—depression, irritability, tears. The better you prepare her, the less apt she is to suffer an embarrassing experience.

Question: Are any of your girlfriends starting to get overly interested in boys? Then you proceed to ask, *Have you found yourself more interested in boys than you used to be?* This may initiate talk about the waves of libido—that is, many girls get a wave of "love sickness" shortly after the beginning of menstruation. At that time they find themselves "prettying up" or dressing to attract boys. Concentration on studies becomes difficult, their grades may suffer, and they will probably be more self-conscious in school and more easily embarrassed around boys than previously. Explaining this probably won't change anything for your daughter, but it will settle two issues: (1) it will explain to her the nature of the forces going on inside her; and (2) it will let her know that you understand. Be sure to clarify that menstruation is part of nature's process in preparing her for maturity.

Question: Do you know what "turns boys on"? Most innocent girls have no idea that tight-fitting sweaters over a shapely emerging bustline is a visual turn-on to boys, as are tight-fitting designer jeans, sexually provocative movements, and skimpy swimsuits.

Some Christian women and their daughters are very naïve about what boys find stimulating. Our Lord declared that if a man looks on a woman to lust after her, he is committing adultery in his mind (Matthew 5:28). This is the time to explain to your daughter that her body can be a symbol of femininity that ennobles men or a symbol of lust that inflames and causes them to stumble spiritually. She may object to the idea that she is "her brother's keeper," but even that becomes an opportunity for you to explain that godly women are modest women. Most innocent girls are confused about the thin line between modest femininity and flirtatious provocativeness. Be sure to discuss with her Paul's advice to all Christians: "Therefore, if what I eat causes my brother to fall into sin, I will never eat meat again, so that I will not cause him to fall" (1 Corinthians 8:13).

Question: Are you aware of the sexual stimulus you give a boy when you touch him? Sometime in her early development every girl should realize that boys develop a sensitivity to female touch before girls realize it. Explain to her that a mature woman's breasts are very sensitive and are used in married lovemaking as a means of sexual arousal. But in some girls, that sensitivity does not begin as soon as the breasts develop, so if a girl is not careful she can inadvertently arouse a boy simply by bumping or rubbing against him.

Question: Are you aware of how the sex drive in a boy

takes place and what arouses it? This may be the means of explaining to your daughter how males function so she can cooperate with nature and not let her body be a cause for sexual fantasy or lust.

Question: *Do you talk about sex with boys?* There seems to be an increasing tendency for people of both sexes to talk openly about this very private subject. Such cross-sexual conversation is cultivated today under the guise of freedom of expression and "openness." I believe this is harmful—not because sex is shameful, but because it is private and is stimulating to both sexes. Such conversation should be saved until marriage and limited to one's partner.

Question: *Have you ever had sexually amorous feelings?* Introduce this question when you think your daughter has been inadvertently exposed via TV, a book, or a movie to sexually suggestive material. It is important that she analyze her feelings. This might be a good time to explain to her "the cycle of a woman" in relation to her monthly period. Your daughter will find that she is generally more affectionate during certain times of the month. She needs to understand the nature of this feeling and its relation to her fertility cycle.

Question: *Are any of the girls your age sexually active?* This might be followed with, *Do your girlfriends talk much about sexual activity?* You need to be aware of your daughter's view of this issue and the status of her moral values. She also needs to know your family rules on dating (see chapter 8) and be held to them.

Question: *Do you know any girls who got pregnant before marriage?* Ask her how she thinks the girl felt and what she should do with the baby. You might also address the current fad of girls getting pregnant deliberately. You might inquire whether she feels this is fair to the child. Let your daughter talk freely without your becoming judgmental. If you automatically declare "what's right," you are apt to shut the conversational door. Don't be upset if she ventures an off-the-wall answer to shock you. Try to respect her opinion, and keep asking questions: *Do you think. . . ?* or *How do you feel about. . . ?*

Question: Have you or any of the girls you go around with heard the old fable that boys like to use after a girl arouses him—that if she doesn't have sex with him, he will be injured physically or psychologically? Even though your daughter would be disobedient to your dating rules if she did get a boy that worked up, she should know that the "stone ache" a boy gets is a physical phenomenon that has no lasting effect. More than anything else, it should show her that she is playing with fire.

Explain that physical intimacy was intended by God to prepare married couples for intercourse, and point out that many "friendship rapes" are caused by boys who get overheated, lose control of their lust, and use their superior force to overpower a girl. The fact that she never intended it to "go all the way" does not lessen the fact that she has lost her virtue, exposed herself to pregnancy, and is partially responsible for the unpleasant situation. Many an unhappy marriage has started this way, and numerous broken dreams were similarly ignited by heavy petting that was never intended to get out of control. Your daughter needs to know that the sex drive in both boys and girls between sixteen and twenty-two is nothing to play with. Like any power, it can get out of control.

Question: Do you or girls your age think you must have sex with a boy to keep his interest? Your daughter should know that such reasoning is false. If she must have sex with him to retain his interest, (1) he is primarily absorbed with her body; (2) it will be a short-lived attachment; and (3) a realized need is a *de*motivator. Many women do not understand that the male who refuses to wait until marriage for sex is not worth having. One reason a young woman who is eager to marry has such a difficult time getting a boy to take her to the altar is that she unwisely submits to his needs before marriage.

Question: Can a girl remain a virgin and still be popular? There is strong peer pressure today on high school girls to engage in premarital sex. It takes strong commitment to moral and spiritual values and encouragement from their parents for girls to see that popularity at age sixteen and seventeen is not nearly so important as integrity and character. At certain times in teenagers' lives they might sacrifice almost anything to be popular. They need to realize that some things are more important than popularity, and giving into teenage sex is not one of them. One hopes that your daughter has been trained to demand character and quality in a young man and to recognize that giving into him sexually may create in him a disgust with both her and himself. That will immediately kill her popularity in his eyes.

In addition, your daughter should be alerted to another teenage certainty: boys talk. In fact, they can be expected to brag about their female exploits. They may promise to keep her confidence while they are going "steady," but after they break up the entire school will know she is an "easy mark." Promiscuous girls are only popular for sex, whereas virtuous girls are admired for themselves.

By the time your daughter is seventeen, she may know far more than you realize, and her questions may be heavier than yours. A survey of high school girls revealed that the following questions were paramount in their minds:

- *How do you avoid sex and still keep a boyfriend?*
- *If I turn a boy on, will it harm him physically?*
- *How far can a girl go without getting into trouble?*
- *How does intercourse feel?*
- *How can I tell if I am ready for sex?*
- *What is the best method of birth control?*
- *Is it better to masturbate each other than have premarital sex?*
- *Is it wrong to have oral sex?*
- *Why should I remain a virgin?*

Have you provided your high school daughter with the answers to these questions?

Reasons You Can Give Your Daughter for Waiting

Emotions often dominate the decision-making process between the ages of fifteen and nineteen, but we underestimate our children if we do not realize that logic and reason also enter into their decisions. Since they are bombarded on every side emotionally to have sex before marriage, only their parents, the church, and some responsible adult friends will provide adequate reasons why they should wait. The following list, designed for Christian parents of teenage girls is not exhaustive, but should be representative.

1. *Your body is not your own, but God's.* Young people need to be told that they serve as the central prize in a war for control of their body. On one side God wants to make it holy and keep it that way, which involves not having sex until marriage. He offers a reward in this life and the life to come for those who keep themselves pure. Those who do so have a better chance of love and happiness in marriage, a guarantee of freedom from VD, and eternal reward. On the other hand, Satan wants to use their bodies for sexual violation of the laws of God and fan their emotions to yield to his will. He uses physical attractions while God uses spiritual, and that is probably why so many Christian youth heed Satan's call instead of God's. But as our Lord warned, Satan is a liar. Instead of premarital sex being all pleasure as he promises, it becomes short-term ecstasy and long-term misery. It breeds guilt, fear, and shame and can lead to premarital pregnancy and incurable strains of VD.

Actually, the Christian young person has no option if she has really committed her body to Jesus Christ. The Bible is very clear. If we obey Christ, we keep our bodies pure; if we engage in premarital sex, we disobey God and dishonor Him. Consider these Scriptures:

> Therefore do not let sin reign in your mortal body so that you obey its evil desires. Do not offer the parts of your body to sin, as instruments of wickedness, but rather offer yourselves to God, as those who have been brought from death to life; and

offer the parts of your body to him as instruments of righteousness. For sin shall not be your master, because you are not under the law, but under grace (Romans 6:12–14).

Do not be yoked together with unbelievers. For what do righteousness and wickedness have in common? Or what fellowship can light have with darkness? What harmony is there between Christ and Belial? What does a believer have in common with an unbeliever? What agreement is there between the temple of God and idols? For we are the temple of the living God. As God has said: "I will live with them and walk among them, and I will be their God, and they will be my people. Therefore come out from them and be separate, says the Lord. Touch no unclean thing, and I will receive you. I will be a Father to you, and you will be my sons and daughters, says the Lord Almighty" (2 Corinthians 6:14–18).

Your daughter needs to hear from you what she probably already knows—that God wants to keep her body pure for His use. If she has this principle impressed into her brain, it will help to strengthen her resolve when she is confronted by temptation.

2. *Virtue helps to maintain self-respect.* One of the greatest problems among modern teens is the lack of self-image. What we think about ourselves profoundly influences our view of God, man, the future, and everything else in our lives. Once a girl violates her virtue, she loses self-respect, making it difficult to come to grips with who she is and thus retarding self-acceptance.

3. *When it's gone, it's gone.* No girl ever became promiscuous until she lost her virtue. Once virginity is gone, however, a powerful spiritual and psychological reason for refusing to engage in premarital sex has also vanished. It is natural for a virgin to want to tell the man she marries that she has saved herself exclusively for him.

4. *Virginity helps you to learn self-control.* The girl who does not gain sexual self-control will probably have a difficult time developing self-control in other matters of life, includ-

ing food, finances, academics, and work. Sex is such a major concern of life that self-mastery is absolutely essential.

5. *Promiscuity usually leads to unwed pregnancy.* Every mother of a teenage girl worries today about the possibility that her daughter could get pregnant prior to marriage. No single event can affect a teen's life and family more critically than this. It creates the ultimate disturbance in a family's life, and it probably means that her life will never again be the same. All her dreams of a beautiful church wedding— usually the happiest day of a girl's life—vanish forever.

The most tragic impact of this event is the damage inflicted on the girl. She is confined at a time in life when she craves activity. Adult responsibilities are thrust upon her prematurely. Education will become difficult at best, impossible at worst. She may miss "Mr. Right," and she may have sentenced herself to a lifetime of economic mediocrity because she had not adequately developed her natural skills. This is an exorbitant price to pay for a few rapturous moments.

7. *Your Christian testimony will be destroyed.* It is difficult for a girl to survive an unwed pregnancy without ruining her entire Christian witness. While it is admittedly unjust for boys not to share equally the full impact of the event, Christian unwed women suffer more. This one act and its natural consequences can undo a positive lifetime testimony.

8. *VD is a risk.* Venereal disease has always been with us, confirming that promiscuity is as old as mankind. The two major strains, syphilis and gonorrhea, have caused untold suffering—birth defects, brain damage, impotence, infertility, and other human miseries. But promiscuity has increased so much in recent years that two new strains, Herpes Simplex II and AIDS, have arrived on the scene as incurable maladies. More will be said about these in the last chapter, and at this point it is sufficient to note that they are

having a frightening effect on sexual patterns. Millions of people have forsaken promiscuity out of fear. This same fear ought to motivate young women to maintain virtue.

A nurse friend of mine has treated a beautiful twenty-nine-year-old prostitute for numerous sores in her mouth resulting from genital herpes. This incurable victim of her own sin was once some mother's virtuous daughter. She knows she will never become a mother, for if she did give birth to a child, more than likely it would come into the world with herpes.

9. *A hasty marriage becomes likely.* A friend told me, "There is a family in our church that I wish could have read this a year ago. Their fifteen-year-old daughter married the seventeen-year-old boy who impregnated her with twins. Now they live in her parents' home, and the boy won't work." Is that the lifestyle those parents had planned for their fifteen-year-old? You can't keep your daughter from ruining her life through premarital sex but you can try. An ounce of prevention (parental sex education) is always worth a pound of cure. Whether to marry the teenage father is a subject in itself, which we will consider in chapter 10. I would observe that the odds of such a marriage working are about two or three times less than if they had waited and she were not pregnant. The unhappiness such young people create for themselves in a premature marriage is incalculable.

God meant children to be a blessing. A hasty teenage marriage as a result of promiscuity usually creates a hindrance instead.

10. *Once begun, teenage sex is difficult to stop.* Once teens begin to have sex, it is all but impossible for them to stop except by breaking off their relationship. The ensuing obsession prevents a couple from getting to know each other on any other level, and unwed pregnancy is almost inevitable. If the truth were known, only a small percentage of couples who engage in teenage sex eventually marry.

11. *A teenage girl risks cancer of the cervix.* The very nature of a girl's body seems to indicate that God never intended for her to have sex at a young age. Dr. Rhoda Lorand, a New York psychiatrist, points out that girls who engage in sex prior to the age of eighteen have an incidence of cancer of the cervix several times greater than those who do not. She concludes that nature built in a protective device for mature women to offset the introduction of the male organ that could bring foreign matter and germs into her vagina. Before age eighteen a woman does not have that immunity; consequently, it is reasonable to conclude that God did not intend very young girls to have sex at all.

These are some of the reasons you can share with your daughter to save the flower of her sexuality for marriage. Let me emphasize again that informed parents are the best sex educators in their children's lives. It is no longer optional; it is a matter of moral survival. We must arm our sons or daughters with all the information they need to make the important decisions in life. Next to the spiritual dimension, nothing affects them more than their sexuality.

A rule of thumb for parentally guided sex education: Start early, be accurate, answer all questions honestly to the best of your ability, maintain an open relationship, and offer a good example of real love between partners.

7

Protecting Our Children From Sexual Abuse

THE MOST WIDESPREAD sexual sin to surface in the eighties is the sexual abuse of children. Every responsible sex counselor I know has been amazed at the frequency with which it occurs in our society. A survey of eight hundred college students indicated that 19 percent of the young women and 9 percent of the men had been sexually abused as children.

Rising statistics could mean that the problem is getting worse, or it may mean we are only talking more openly about it, which has freed more adults to confess their childhood experiences. The $8 billion pornography business and the filthy movies shown on cable TV have done nothing for chastity in the home. According to one government authority, current statistics suggest that 25 percent of all girls will be molested by the time they are thirteen years old, one-third by the time they are seventeen. Never has there been a more urgent need than today for parents to protect their children sexually.

Whereas child molestation by strangers is a frighteningly dangerous trend, outsiders are by no means the only ones whom children must fear. Many children are sexually abused by members of their own families. The breakdown of the family in American society aggravates potential problems. One vulnerable situation is the stepfamily in which a man has a blossoming teenage stepdaughter who is more sexually attractive than her mother, or a young girl is too weak to fight off an older stepbrother.

Depression-producing guilt and the loss of self-respect are frequently the result of teenage girls and young women being sexually molested as children. In addition, they often become angry, frigid, or promiscuous; some resort to lesbianism. Many molested girls grow up and marry beneath their potential because of this guilt and shame, thus making their entire lives miserable as a result of someone else's sin.

GIRLS—THE PRINCIPAL VICTIMS

Girls are victims of sexual abuse in much greater numbers than boys. I become angry just thinking of a man sexually violating a child. My emotional thermometer rises sharply when I learn of a girl's own father perpetrating the deed. I am almost embarrassed to recount the first such case I faced in the counseling room. A beautiful fifteen-year-old came to ask how she could make her father stop demanding sex from her without letting him know that she had confided her dilemma to me. "If he knew I told you, he would kill me," she said. When I insisted that she should tell her mother, she replied, "I already did, but she is afraid she will lose him if she doesn't let him."

These were not pagans; they were members of my church. I was able to stop this molestation, but two years later the girl became promiscuous and pregnant. After all, she had no virtue to protect because of her father. Years later this man died a long and painful death. I couldn't help thinking that he may have suffered the just reward of his deeds.

Little girls and teenagers are especially vulnerable to

sexual abuse by men—in some cases their own brothers. Usually they are physically forced or seduced, then threatened into silence with revenge if they tell anyone. Sometimes, when a victim is driven by guilt or anger to disclose the situation, the mother doesn't believe the sordid tale or refuses to face the truth.

What kind of a man or boy would sexually molest a helpless girl? Here are some of their characteristics:

- A sexually obsessed male who reads pornographic literature or views sexually explicit movies;
- An alcoholic or heavy drinker who loses his self-control but not his sex drive when drinking;
- An insecure man who is afraid of being rejected by a woman his own age and thus picks on a child;
- An infantile man who cannot relate to adults but spends much time with children;
- Men married to overpowering and dominant women who stifle them sexually, so that they turn to their own children or stepchildren, who are more submissive;
- Undisciplined men who fail at all they set out to do but find that sexual conquest of a child gives them a much-needed feeling of power;
- Brainwashed victims of our humanistic society who actually talk themselves into thinking that it is good for children to become sexually active early in life and that adult-child sex is a "loving experience" that is beneficial to the child.

Such individuals are sin-sick. Our children must be protected from them.

WHY THE INCREASE IN CHILD MOLESTATION?

We have already touched on possible causes for the increase in child molestation, but it is helpful to deal with them here in greater detail. There are three reasons for doing this: (1) That we might store them in our minds so that if we encounter these conditions, we can be wary. In this day and age, all parents should keep mentally attuned to any sign that their children are in danger and act to protect them at all costs; (2) That we might become active in the event our community or state moves to effect legal change in dealing with child sexual abuse; (3)   as Christians we should be concerned about protecting the lives of all children. To do so, we must initiate legislative reform. Pornographers and movie makers have already demonstrated that they are irresponsible in the kinds of programming they present. They must be controlled by legislation, which will be enacted only when enough morally committed people rise up and demand it.

We have never heard more about the tragedy of sexual abuse of children than we do today. From the church to the government, everyone is concerned. Some have raised their voices on television to warn about the alarming increase in this problem. Unfortunately, they rarely speak to the true causes, perhaps because they don't understand them.

The following are my suggestions as to what causes adults—principally men—to abuse children sexually. Until these social conditions change, we will continue to experience an increasing number of innocent children assaulted in their own homes each year.

1. *The expanding publication of pornographic litera-ture.* This year the organized crime-controlled pornography industry will do at least $8 billion worth of business. According to Bruce Taylor, vice-president of Citizens for Decency Through Law, the Mafia launders millions of dollars of drug and prostitution money through pornography bookstores, peepshows, and X-rated theaters, so we cannot know precisely how big the porn business really is. But we are certain that it is a multibillion-dollar industry that can wield enormous power in our courts and keep the wrong kinds of politicians in office.

I consider this form of mental depravity the number one cause of the alarming increase in child molestation and assault. I know of cases where teenage brothers read their father's pornographic magazines and became so emotionally overheated that they raped their own sisters. Only God knows how often this occurs, for shame and fear keep many girls from reporting the crime.

But the testimonies of women indicate that the problem has existed for years and will continue to accelerate as long as corrupt minds have easy access to pornography. Pornography is to the mind and emotions of men what gasoline is to fire; it has become the single most inflammatory force for evil in our society. Until judges stop heeding the cry of attorneys who appeal to the First Amendment as their defense and start to protect our children, the problem will remain an unquenchable inferno.

2. *Filthy or suggestive movies and TV programs.* These are working their way into the homes of our country on both network and cable TV, inciting depraved men and immature but sexually capable boys. If television networks continue to degenerate at the current rate, we can expect an "anything goes" type of morality to be brought right into 99 percent of the American homes that currently have television sets. I predict that there will be a competition between the networks, cable, and Home Box Office to see who can offer the most depraved fare—and the movie makers will serve as chefs. Either this sexually inflammatory material must be halted by the courts, or an increasing number of innocent girls will fall victim to molestation and abuse.

3. *Working wives who leave children untended in the home for long periods of time, offering temptations to fathers or brothers to indulge in child molestation.* Currently 60 percent of the married women in the United States work outside the home. It is estimated that by the turn of the century the number will approach 75 percent. That leaves millions of children alone and vulnerable or taken to day-care centers. As we have learned from the media, day-care centers are not universally the protectors of children they were once thought to be.

4. *Divorce and remarriage.* More than 1.3 million couples received divorces in 1984. Of these, almost one million will remarry. This offers a strong temptation to stepbrothers and stepfathers, particularly if they are pornography users or TV addicts.

5. *Drugs and alcohol.* Alcohol breaks down a person's normal reserve and inflames dangerous passions that can easily be translated into the sexual abuse of children.

6. *Indiscreet parents.* Some families' living quarters do not contribute to privacy for parents today, and many people have lost their sense of discretion. Watching parents indulge in intercourse can lead brothers and sisters to experiment. Any sexual exhibitionism in the home may have an adverse effect on the safety of our little girls.

7. *A general breakdown in moral values.* In times of temptation it is good to be fortified by moral resolve. This comes only by emphasizing the traditional moral values of the Bible. Sunday schools and Christian schools are doing an excellent job of this with about 45 percent of American youth. But the 43 million public school children who do not imbibe these values at home or in church will grow up without such moral resolve, because public schools have all but abandoned responsibility for teaching traditional values or they directly assault them.

As long as these and other causes of child molestation remain, we can expect a steady increase in the problem. If we do not confront the problem through legislation or experience a moral and spiritual revival, I predict that by the twenty-first century the percentage of female victims of sexual molestation under age seventeen will increase to more than 50 percent in the United States.

The family frustration, guilt, isolation, anger and intense unhappiness caused by the abusers, by their victims, and by those who can't or won't do anything to stop it cannot be calculated. Imagine the desperation of the working mother who came to me because she felt "trapped in a no-win second marriage." Her husband of five years was becoming disinterested in her sexually, was drinking heavily, and had begun to look lustily at his fourteen-year-old stepdaughter. Outraged at her treatment, the girl was complaining to her mother that she "can't stand the way he paws me." This working mother, now pregnant and financially dependent on her husband, was terrified by what her husband might do to the daughter, "the one person in my life I love most."

God meant the home to be a child's haven of protection from the evils of society. Because of the humanistic philosophy that permeates our media, government, and educators today, that evil society is infiltrating the home and assaulting our children.

The home environment, however, is not the only place where child sexual abuse takes place. In the early eighties, national media focused attention on widespread exploitation outside the home. Numerous revelations of child pornography rings operating in certified day-care centers suddenly hit the headlines and TV talk shows.

Kee MacFarlane, director of the Child Sexual Abuse Diagnostic and Treatment Center of the Children's Institute International in Los Angeles, believes there is a nationwide network of "child predators" who have opened day-care centers so they will have access to young children. In her testimony before a congressional committee, Miss MacFarlane made this statement:

> I believe that we're dealing with a conspiracy, an organized operation of child predators designed to prevent detection. The preschool, in such a case, serves as a ruse for a larger unthinkable network of crimes against children. If such an operation involves child pornography or the selling of children, as is frequently alleged, it may have greater financial, legal and community resources at its disposal than those attempting to expose it.[1]

It is feared by many responsible observers that the problem of day-care abuse is far more prevalent than most people believe. Parents must be more careful whom they permit to care for their children.

THE DAMAGE TO CHILDREN

Children who are sexually abused often suffer irreparable emotional, physical, and spiritual damage. They may suffer lacerated genitals and rectal damage; they face a higher than normal risk of cervical cancer in later years. Cliff Linedecker, author of *Children in Chains,* which is an exposé of child pornography, prostitution, and sexual abuse, tells the story of a fourteen-year-old boy in Chicago who was placed in a foster home. His state-appointed guardian turned out to be a pedophile (child molester) who regularly forced him to engage in oral sex. After this youngster fled to the police for protection, it was discovered that he had gonorrhea of the throat.

The emotional damage caused by child abuse is often irreversible. Cliff Linedecker has observed, "Children who are used sexually by adults or who are seduced, enticed, or forced to pose for pornography are left almost inevitably with severe psychological scarring that can never be erased.[2] Some of these emotional scars are feelings of worthlessness, guilt, betrayal, rage, powerlessness, and distrust. As adults, victims of child sexual abuse are often unable to maintain normal relationships with other people. They feel unwanted, dirty, and useless.

The Texas Department of Human Resources (Select Committee on Child Pornography, 1978) listed seventeen short-term side effects of child sexual abuse: (1) Regressive behavior; (2) delinquent behavior; (3) sexual promiscuity; (4) poor peer relationships; (5) unwillingness to participate in physical and/or recreational activities; (6) running away; (7) drug or alcohol abuse; (8) confusion; (9) depression;

(10) anxiety; (11) suspicion; (12) bad dreams; (13) restlessness; (14) personal behavior inconsistent with prior behavioral patterns; (15) unexplained medical problems; (16) learning disabilities; (17) self-mutilation.[3]

A PROFILE OF CHILD MOLESTERS

Two stories related to child molesting appeared in the *San Diego Union* on November 18, 1984. The headlines read "Alleged Sex Offender to Stand Trial" and "Man Gets 10 Years for Molesting Boy." In one case a fifty-six-year-old man was charged with "multiple counts of child molesting, having unlawful sex with minors, oral copulation, pandering, soliciting lewd and lascivious acts with a child, contributing to the delinquency of minors and child pornography." In the other case a man was given a ten-year jail sentence on charges relating to a young boy in a voluntary social service program.

In June 1984 the *Los Angeles Times* carried an article headlined "Minister Who Committed Sex Case to Be Freed." This told the story of a pastor who had recently been released from Patton State Mental Hospital, where he had been confined for six years as a "mentally disordered sex offender." He was serving as the principal of a Christian high school when he was arrested on charges of sexually abusing several teenage boys.

What does a sex molester look like? Dr. Bruce Gross, acting director of the USC Institute of Psychiatry, Law and Behavioral Science, has seen more than a thousand child molesters in the last twelve years. His description: "It's impossible to identify them. They look like the typical person in the community." A youth pastor, boys club director, airport executive, priest, security officer, boy scout leader, elementary schoolteacher—all these kinds of people have been convicted of child molestation in California in recent years.

Molesters do not fit the stereotypical image of the "dirty old man" (although 90 percent of the people arrested for molestation are men). They are vastly different. They do not fit into any narrow ethnic, social, or economic categories, although patterns can be discerned among other character- istics. It is known that the majority of molesters are not strangers to the children; they are trusted friends, relatives, community leaders, and other authority figures.

Cliff Linedecker cautions,

> The child pornographer or panderer of today is more likely to be sophisticated, mobile, educated, and wealthy. Often he is a pillar of his community and is respected for his involvement in youth-oriented activities such as scouting for boys or girls, church-sponsored programs, summer camps, and other ac- cepted activities for building character in the young. Several men connected to child pornography and child prostitution rings are millionaires.[4]

The molester who is known to a child is seldom bent on violence. Stunted emotionally, he is simply displaying child- like feelings and attitudes. Dr. Shirley O'Brien, writing in *Child Pornography,* describes the pedophile as someone who is emotionally immature.

> Some men with pedophiliac tendencies do marry and have children. Even so, they may still exhibit these immature characteristics and remain sexually inadequate. If pressured or rejected by his spouse, he may seek gratification with a child. He will seek someone who is accepting, someone who will do his bidding and not make fun of him.[5]

The pedophile actually believes that he "loves" the child with whom he has sexual relations. He woos the youngster much as a man courts a woman, and he photographs the child because he knows the relationship cannot last forever. Frequently he trades pictures with his friends, who operate in an informal network; some of the photographs may eventually end up in pornographic magazines.

Molesters As Victims of Abuse

There is considerable evidence that adult molesters of children were themselves victims of sexual abuse as youngsters. A. Nicholas Groth, a clinical psychologist and director of the sex-offender program at the Connecticut Correctional Institution, has worked with molesters for eighteen years. He has identified a consistent pattern: unstable, unsettled families; lack of consistent or fair discipline in the home; and abuse or neglect at home. Groth found "evidence of some form of sexual trauma in the life histories of about one-third of the offenders he worked with. This statistic was significant when compared with the finding that only about one-tenth of adult male nonoffenders report similar victimization in their lives."[6]

A Dangerous New Breed of Molester

Dr. Bruce Gross of USC is alarmed about what he calls a new breed of child molester. He is concerned with men who have been convicted and are now out of jail. According to Gross, if such people continue to molest children, "the likelihood of them killing their victim is extremely high."[7] With a conviction already behind them, these men fear they will face longer jail sentences if they are arrested again and therefore can rationalize killing children just to destroy potential witnesses.

PROTECTING OUR CHILDREN

The following list enumerates methods commonly used by child molesters—especially men who are strangers to the victim. This list was developed by Kenneth Wooden, executive director of the National Coalition for Children's Justice. It is good for us as parents to discuss these with our children.

1. *Affection/Love.* Most child molestations and murders are committed by someone who is known by the child or is a member of the family.

2. *Assistance.* Molesters often approach a child asking for help of some kind: directions to a popular landmark, nearby restaurant, or school; assistance in finding a lost puppy; aid in carrying an armload of packages to a car.

3. *Authority.* Because children have respect for authority, molesters take advantage of them by dressing as police officers, clergy, or firemen.

4. *Bribery.* This is one of the oldest ruses. Children may be offered toys, candy, or other rewards.

5. *Ego/Fame.* Sometimes children are promised a modeling job, the chance to compete in a beauty contest, or the opportunity to star in a television commercial.

6. *Emergency.* The emergency lure is designed to disarm, confuse, and worry a child.

7. *Games and Fun.* With this enticement, seemingly innocent play often leads to intimate bodily contact.

8. *Jobs.* Older children can be attracted by an offer of high-paying or interesting jobs.

9. *Threats or Fear.* Some molesters use threats of violence, flashing guns or knives before the victim.

By discussing these tactics with our children, we can reduce the risks of their falling victim to sexual abuse. Because as many as 100,000 to 500,000 children are molested each year, it is essential that we provide our children with the information they need to avoid becoming victims.

One of the most sensitive approaches to child abuse has been produced by William Katz, head of the Christian Society for the Prevention of Cruelty to Children. The "Little Ones" educational program includes *Protecting Your Children From Sexual Assault,* which is a parent teaching guide, and *Little Ones Activity Book,* a coloring book for children. By leading children through the activity book, we can provide them with a thorough understanding of God's love, the importance of privacy, and their right to say no to someone who attempts to touch them. The activity book takes children through a series of lessons on "yes" and "no" touching. It shows them when it is appropriate for someone to hug or show affection. Then it teaches them to resist the kind of touching that violates their privacy. Information on the "Little Ones" materials can be obtained from the Christian Society for the Prevention of Cruelty to Children, 8200 Grand Avenue South, Bloomington, MN 55420.

Keeping Alert to Signs

We must keep alert for signs of possible child molestation. What do we look for?

1. Unusual marks, bruises, or reddening around the anus or genitals.

2. Personality modification. Abrupt changes in behavior may indicate sexual problems. Dr. Shirley O'Brien has warned, "If a child's personality seems to change overnight and the pattern persists, it is a signal that something is wrong."[8]

3. Depression. Has the child suddenly become chronically depressed for no apparent reason?

4. Secretiveness. Has the child suddenly become sneaky about his activities? Has he been caught lying about where he spends his time?

5. Language. Is the child demonstrating a sophisticated knowledge of sexual terms or activities?

6. Material goods. Has the child recently acquired toys, clothing, or money whose source cannot be accounted for? Bribery could be the cause.

Teaching our children about sexual abuse must become a central feature of our sex education program. To ignore the dangers posed by child molesters is to leave our children vulnerable to abuse and exploitation. We should encourage them to tell us whenever they encounter a situation they don't quite understand. As the rate of female child molestation continues to rise, it becomes essential that we safeguard our daughters in particular by opening the conversational door to the subject. It may be difficult for a small child to talk to her mother about this delicate subject, but we must make sure our daughters know that if anyone ever touches their private parts, they must come and tell us. This communication removes the guilt feelings so common in children and helps us to preserve our children's innocence. A child's assurance of freedom to open a conversation about this subject at any time is our best means of protection.

HOW TO REACT IF A CHILD HAS BEEN MOLESTED

If one of our children has been molested, we must first realize that he needs our reassurance that we will take care of him and continue to love him. Often a child who has been victimized will feel like the guilty party. We must let the victim know that everything will be all right and that no one will blame him for what has happened.

We should go slow in trying to find out exactly what happened and who did it. Don't rush the child. He will be experiencing conflicting emotions and desperately needs our love and respect. Also, he may feel that he is betraying a "friend" by divulging details, for it is standard procedure for a pedophile to swear a child to secrecy. Because we train our children to keep promises, they may become confused when we ask them to break a promise.

If there is physical evidence on the child's clothing or body, let it stand. For instance, we should not wash the child's genitals until he has a medical examination, lest we destroy evidence. Once we have determined to our own satisfaction that the child has indeed been molested, we should contact the local police department. We will be directed to an appropriate medical facility.

We must be careful to keep the channels of communication open. We must love our children, pay attention to them, and continually emphasize our willingness to discuss sexual matters with them. Most important, we must pray for them daily.

The apostle Paul describes further means for protection in Ephesians 6:13–18.

> Therefore put on the full armor of God, so that when the day of evil comes, you may stand your ground, and after you have done everything, to stand. Stand firm then, with the belt of truth buckled round your waist, with the breastplate of righteousness in place, and with your feet fitted with the readiness that comes from the gospel of peace. In addition to all this, take up the shield of faith, with which you can extinguish all the flaming arrows of the evil one. Take the helmet of salvation and the sword of the Spirit, which is the word of God. And pray in the Spirit on all occasions with all kinds of prayers and requests. With this in mind, be alert and always keep on praying for all the saints.

8

Guidelines for Dating

DATING IS AN EXCITING experience not only for a teenager, but also for Father and Mother. Some parents find it traumatic; others consider it an enjoyable part of raising their children.

The dating stage of life usually catches both teenagers and their parents unprepared. Young people have little idea what their parents expect of them, and parents are not always in agreement with each other. That's a formula for disaster. We prepare our children for school, Sunday school, birthdays, Christmas, swimming lessons, and almost every other event in life. Why do we fail to lay a proper foundation for dating? Beverly and I have discovered that if a strategic plan of action is instituted for the first child, it is relatively simple to get younger brothers and sisters to accept the same standards. But if parents strike out with the first, they may lose the ball game with the others.

Dating arouses fear in many parents for several reasons. First, it represents a giant step toward independence. Parents seldom accompany the dating couple; consequently, they lose a large measure of control when teens go out for two to four hours at a time. Second, some parents have not learned to trust their children, and dating accentuates that lack of trust. Third, they have not prepared guidelines in advance; thus, their fears become exaggerated.

Beverly and I have had the privilege of using our guidelines for dating on ten children—four of our own, plus six missionary children whose parents sent them to live with us for their junior or senior years of high school. Whenever we accepted teenagers of missionaries, it was on the condition that they accept our dating standards. Although we had confrontations at times, with both the missionaries' children and our own, dating was basically a pleasurable time for all of us.

STANDARDS FOR DATING

The following list offers the standards we have developed through the years. They are not perfect, but they worked for us and have been used by thousands of families who have attended our Family Life Seminars. At times your popularity as a parent will drop if you enforce standards such as these; but if you lack guidelines, both you and your teenagers will live to regret it. Popularity will be meaningless then.

1. *Dating is for fifteen-year-olds and over.* Reserving dating for this age bracket is no problem for boys. Many of them are not interested in girls until later, or couldn't afford to date even if they were interested. Girls are different. As we have noted, they mature earlier than boys both physically and socially. Therefore they are often eager to start dating earlier. Boys their own age are frequently disinterested or unappealing, so don't be surprised if they want to date older boys. That, of course, presents a special set of problems.

Although fifteen is a recommended age for dating, this should not eliminate young people from enjoying each other's company in group activities—church youth outings, camp, sports events, or parties. But official dating, when a boy comes to a girl's home to take her out, should be reserved until the fifteenth birthday.

2. *Date only Christians.* One cardinal principle is clearly specified in the Word of God: "Be ye not unequally yoked together with unbelievers" (2 Corinthians 6:14 KJV). Dating is a yoke of fellowship that can eventually lead to marriage. We can help our young people avoid the emotional trauma of ever having to decide "Should I marry this unsaved person with whom I am very much in love or should we break up?" by refusing to let them go out with such people in the first place. Remember, our sons and daughters will seldom get seriously involved with someone they do not date.

This standard may draw a few tears when a teenage girl is forbidden to keep company with the handsome high school quarterback with whom she is infatuated, but it will forestall a calamity later. The apostle Paul may have had this in mind when he wrote, "Bad company corrupts good morals" (1 Corinthians 15:35 NASB). We will find that any young person who does not come from a home that shares our moral values will have a harmful and even "corrupting" influence on our sons or daughters.

Through the years Beverly and I have watched fine, dedicated Christians lose their children, whom they dearly loved, because they did not establish this standard. We have recently prayed and cried with several who lived to regret it. Two daughters, married at eighteen and divorced at nineteen, broke the hearts of their parents and deeply troubled the waters of early adulthood.

3. *Schedule a predating interview with Father.* When a young man dates your daughter, it is serious business because he is going out with one of your most treasured possessions. If a person borrowed your car or boat, you would set some guidelines for its use. It is even more important when a young man "borrows" your daughter. This may frighten some prospects away, but they represent the group you want your daughter to avoid. Any boy who lacks the courage to look a girl's father in the eye when asking permission has no business dating her.

This interview gives Father the opportunity to do four things. First, he can see for himself whether the young man is really a Christian (hearsay testimonies aren't always valid). Second, he can check the boy's motivation. Does he have goals or plans for his life according to his age level, or is your daughter his only immediate objective? Third, he can clearly lay down the guidelines they are to follow. Don't expect your daughter to do this; expecting her to do so would be embarrassing for her, and something might be missed in the transmission. Fourth, he can size up the young man's home life. If the person loves and respects his parents, you can discern more readily what to expect in your relationships with him. The converse is also true.

When your son wants to date a Christian girl, it is somewhat easier for you to share with him your guidelines. If he dates the same girl two or three times and you don't know her personally, have him bring her along to a family outing or arrange an interview involving both you and your spouse. (I suggest that Mother be involved in this interview because fathers can be misled. It takes a woman to evaluate a woman, particularly when her son is involved.)

Bill Gothard teaches at his seminars that guidelines for dating, including an interview with Father, are very important. This has fortified our procedure and in recent years has made the process much easier for Christian young people to accept.

4. *All dates must be approved in advance.* Until young people get acquainted with you and your standards, don't let them manipulate you into quick approval of some type of activity that you do not favor. We made it clear to our teens that approved dating could include all church activities and outings, chaperoned parties, sports events, and special occasions they wished to request. The don't-bother-to-ask list included movies, dances, unchaperoned private parties, and any activity where drinking took place.

5. *Until high school graduation, only double dating is*

permitted. Probably the one requirement our teenagers objected to most was double dating with another Christian couple. There is safety in numbers—not much, but some. The main reason for this, however, is to force the teenagers to make plans in advance and to avoid long periods of time when they can drift into "heavy couple talk." Under a wave of libido and the romance of the moment, young people can easily make premature love statements and commitments they don't really mean. The presence of another couple greatly reduces this possibility, though it does not eliminate it altogether.

It is admittedly difficult at times to organize a double date, so to compensate for our stringent rules, we went out of our way to make the family car available to our son whenever his request was legitimate. If your son has wheels, it usually isn't difficult for him to find a friend with whom to double date, if he really wants to.

6. *Absolutely no parking.* Mount Helix (or the lover's vantage point in your community) may be an exciting place to "view the lights of the city," but it is not an ideal environment for avoiding youthful temptations. At this stage of life, touching the opposite sex is exciting, stimulating, and dangerous. We view dating as a time of fun and social fellowship, not a test of self-control.

One of our children irritably protested, "Dad, I get the feeling you don't trust us!" I replied, "You're right. I don't trust you, myself, or anyone else who makes provision for the flesh." You may ask, "Didn't your children ever park during their dating years?" We aren't so naïve as to think they didn't, but if they did, we wanted it clearly understood that it violated our rules. One girl admitted, "Whenever I was tempted to park while on a date with a boy, I was always afraid my father might rise up out of the back seat."

7. *Never go to a home or confined quarters without a responsible adult in attendance.* In a former time the automobile was the primary arena in which girls lost their

virtue or became pregnant (particularly at drive-in theaters). That day is past. Because automakers have miniaturized cars and popularized bucket seats, one would have to be a contortionist to have sex in today's most popular vehicles.

Moreover, homes untended by working adults are fully accessible today, providing an environment much more conducive to "making out" and much more inciting to sexual relations than any car. Such places should be expressly off limits even for the most trustworthy teens. The Bible instructs us "to abstain from every appearance of evil" (1 Thessalonians 5:22 NKJV). Two teens of the opposite sex in an untended house may not misbehave, but their unsupervised presence together could ruin their reputations and should be expressly forbidden.

8. *No undue public show of affection.* Love is beautiful to both teens and adults, but public demonstrations of affection that border on suggestiveness are harmful to a person's testimony and may imply moral license to others. The Christian community applauds teenagers who love each other but have enough self-respect not to maul one another in public. Proper dating should not detract from a young person's testimony or spiritual growth; besides, open expressions of affection today may prove embarrassing later, should the interest in that person evaporate.

9. *Avoid all petting, caressing, or other physical expressions of affection that lead to sexual arousal.* This is perhaps the toughest rule of all. But after all, what is petting? In marriage we call it "foreplay," and one of its purposes is to prepare a husband and wife for intercourse. Only the most naïve fail to realize that the same preparations occur in the unmarried who engage in heavy petting. Most initial sex experiences before marriage occur as a result of this activity, though they were probably not the original intentions of either party.

The problem with sexual arousal is that most people experience a "point of no return." No one can predict it, and because of the highs and lows of libido, a person is at times powerless to control his sexual drive after it is brought to a peak. The time to control it is before arousal. Sexual passions are not evil when reserved for the sanctity of marriage. Unmarried teenagers should avoid that kind of temptation.

Because sexual arousal is more exciting than any other activity, the couple who indulge this pastime become dissatisfied with other worthwhile and meaningful dating activities. Once experienced, petting seems to take precedence over everything else and usually claims an increasing amount of time. Heavy petting usually leads to intercourse. If marriage must be delayed between two lovers, then petting should also be postponed. In fact, to avoid spiritual and moral difficulties, couples should reserve it exclusively for marriage.

One reason for the high divorce rate today is that young people have engaged in such extensive petting that they know each other almost exclusively on the level of physical intimacy. This often blinds them to traits that may have discouraged matrimony had they not been so preoccupied. There is plenty of time for lovemaking after marriage. Until then, young people should be encouraged to participate in activities that will acquaint them with each other in various ways and provide them rich hours of pleasure. Such activities will be neglected if they have to compete with sexual arousal. Young people should be urged to enjoy the freedom of youth, a fleeting period of time that need not be encumbered by the responsibilities and activities of adulthood.

The most detrimental part of all is that sexual intimacy keeps teenagers from hearing the Holy Spirit as He speaks to them about committing themselves to a vocation of lifelong service to our Lord.

10. *Curfew should be set at 11:00 P.M. for girls, 11:30 for boys* (with approved exceptions). Aside from certain well-chaperoned functions we knew in advance would last later than 10:30 P.M., we expected our girls home at 11:00 and our

boys at 11:30. (This allowed time for our son to escort two girls and another fellow home without missing the curfew.) These deadlines were universally resisted at first and may have been earlier than those set by most parents, but we reasoned that very little wholesome activity occurred in our city after eleven o'clock. The good snack shops close then, and we think teenagers should be home by that time. Admittedly, most parents are more lenient. One of our daughters complained tearfully, "Dad, I'm the only girl in the church that has to be in by eleven." I lovingly reassured her, "I can't help it if the rest of the parents are wrong."

Our son remarked after marriage, "One thing I found embarrassing about our family's dating rules was that all the girls I dated had a later curfew than I did." One girl asked him, "Larry, why are you bringing me home at eleven? I don't have to be in until twelve." If I were setting the guidelines today, I would probably be more lenient—I'd set the curfew at 11:30 for high school seniors.

In spite of the embarrassment and minor problems, we have no regrets. One daughter who often chafed under the curfew commented four months after the birth of her daughter, "Remember those dating rules? We're planning to use the same ones for Jenny when she's old enough to date." Parents have a different perspective than teenagers.

Some parents may not know how to enforce the curfew. Whatever hour you set will usually be considered too early and may be ignored, and this will create conflict between parents and teens. We solved that problem simply by stating that every minute they were late coming home would cost them a fifteen-minute penalty on the next date. One boy brought our daughter home so late that their next date was only one and one-half hours long. They had to cut short their miniature golfing on the seventh hole to make it home on time. But in four years of dating after that, they were late only once, when they had a flat tire on the freeway. Young people need to know that parents will keep their word. When they test your rules, be sure you don't flunk the examination.

Many parents consider these guidelines too stringent and thus decide to "massage the rules." Too often parents decide, "I can trust my children," so they let them establish their own dating standards or give them too much flexibility. In some cases it has worked very well, but in many others we have seen the quality training of early childhood and early adolescence tragically marred by excessive dating freedom. These parents have forgotten the powerful influence of teenagers on each other and the power of the normal teenage libido.

It is tragic when the self-control lessons of childhood are overpowered by these new and exciting drives, confronted when teens are least able to cope with them. In all of life these are the years of greatest emotional instability; thus decisions will often be made on the basis of emotion rather than mind and will. Someone has said, "When the emotion and will are in conflict, the emotions invariably win." This is dangerous, because emotion-based decisions are almost always wrong. It takes a good deal of maturity for anyone to learn that only when the mind and emotions agree is it right to proceed with anything. Even then, the mind should be guided by the Word of God. Solomon counseled, "A wise son makes a father glad, but a foolish son is a grief to his mother" (Proverbs 10:1 NASB). What is true of sons holds true for daughters also.*

Keep in mind that whenever we have to be inflexible in the application of a dating rule, we should take pains to be friendly, loving, and sometimes compensatory. But we must not be too lenient. Our culture has provided teenagers with a custom called dating that was not practiced in biblical times. In those days it was customary for parents to make the choice of their children's partners, which usually precluded teenage dating, promiscuity, and pregnancy out of wedlock. I am not advocating a return to customs of two thousand years

---

*For further discussion of this matter, see Beverly LaHaye, *How to Develop Your Child's Temperament* (Irvine, Calif.: Harvest House, 1977), 108-144.

ago, but parents must not leave such decisions as "Who can I date?" or "What can I do on a date?" or "Where can I go?" or "How late can I stay out?" to teenagers who just a few years before were elementary children. Those decisions, leading to adult responsibilities, are made by teens at their peril. This is one matter that can rightly be labeled "parental guidance required."

Dating can be a delightful experience for both teenagers and their parents. But it will be enjoyed best and longest when we safeguard our teenagers' futures by providing guidelines through this important stage in life and lovingly see to it that they are maintained.

9

Christian Moral Values

A LITTLE MORE than fifty years ago, something happened at Cambridge University that illustrates the modern dilemma of Christian moral values in a hostile culture. A well-known science professor who prided himself on making his lectures interesting to every member of his class discovered one older woman who was bored to death. Upon questioning, he discovered that she was the official chaperone for the women students in his class.

How long has it been since you have heard of chaperones for ladies? Fifty years ago male students were forbidden to set foot in women's dormitories, even to visit their sisters. Today coed dormitories, replete with sexual promiscuity are commonplace. One girl fretted, "I hate to live in the dorm. I never know whom my roommate will bring to spend the night with her."

It is now generally accepted, that "the Christian consensus" that once established the moral values of our nation has been replaced with an "anything goes" or "whatever feels good is permissible" morality. We have already noted today a smaller percentage of young men and women enter marriage as virgins than just twenty years ago. Although there are no official surveys of church young people, unofficial data and personal observations suggest that our high school and college adults are not a great deal different except that they may tend to experience longer courtships and less promiscuity. But their rate of virginity upon entering marriage is frighteningly low.

In a day when almost all liberal educators, psychologists, sociologists, and other framers of public opinion (including TV programmers, rock stars, and Hollywood personalities) advocate free sex and promiscuity, we need to come back to basics—the basics of what God says about human sexuality. That is the duty of the church and the Christian community: to speak out boldly on moral issues when a culture turns its back on that which exists for its benefit.

One of the dangers of television is that it does not advertise the religious bias of those it interviews. Just recently a prominent film star was reflecting on youthful morality. A network's prime time was given to this star who had acted every kind of immoral part imaginable, including prostitute, nymphomaniac, unfaithful wife, and lesbian. Her valueless comments, which hardly improve anyone's morals, coincided with the fact that she was married three times and is currently living with a man out of wedlock.

However, if Jerry Falwell or any other minister of the gospel is interviewed on TV concerning his views, his attitudes are usually presented as "judgmental," "fundamentalist," "right wing," "puritanical," or "passé." An old debate tactic is repeatedly used by the media. If you cannot defeat your opponent with logic, try ridicule, character assassination, or distortion of their views. Until genital herpes and AIDS came into prominence, antimoralists made those who advocated that "sex should be reserved for marriage" sound inhuman and outmoded. Now serious people are taking a new look at the old moral absolutes as a means of ensuring both health and happiness.

Our young people have to make up their minds in the midst of this liberal culture as to which standards will chart the course of their lives, man's or God's. This chapter is a simple presentation of what the Bible teaches about moral values. They are clear, absolute, and unchangeable. Every Christian parent should acquaint his teenagers with God's teachings on this subject; otherwise they will be overly impressed with man's point of view, which usually promotes permissiveness. The Bible teaches, "Happy is the man who does not walk in the counsel of the ungodly" (Psalm 1:1).

The safeguard of implanting God's word is young minds as an antidote to sin and temptation appears in the words of David, "Thy word have I hid in my heart that I might not sin against you" (Psalm 119:11). In the hours of temptation our young people will need all the help they can get. These scriptures will give them that support and encouragement.

ADULTERY AND FORNICATION: ALWAYS FORBIDDEN

Adultery in the Bible means any form of sexual relationship outside of marriage, and it is always prohibited. Consider the following passages.

Old Testament

"You shall not commit adultery" (Exodus 20:14; Deuteronomy 5:18).

"Consecrate yourselves and be holy, because I am the LORD your God. . . .

"If a man commits adultery with another man's wife—with the wife of his neighbor—both the adulterer and adulteress must be put to death.

"If a man sleeps with his father's wife, he had dishonored his father. Both the man and the woman must be put to death; their blood will be on their own heads.

"If a man sleeps with his daughter-in-law, both of them must be put to death. What they have done is a perversion; their blood will be on their own heads.

"If a man lies with a man as one lies with a woman, both of them have done what is detestable. They must be put to death; their blood will be on their own heads" (Leviticus 20:7, 10–13).

These moral laws were given to Israel as they entered the land of Palestine "to preserve life." While we do not advocate putting people to death for adultery, the penalty does indicate the rigor of God's moral laws. Obviously God was serious when He commanded men and women not to use their sexuality outside of marriage. The following proverbs were given after Israel had been in the Promised Land for several hundred years:

"My son, pay attention to my wisdom, listen well to my words of insight, that you may maintain discretion and your lips may preserve knowledge. For the lips of an adulteress drip honey, and her speech is smoother than oil; but in the end she is bitter as gall; sharp as a double-edged sword. Her feet go down to death; her steps lead straight to the grave. She gives no thought to the way of life; her paths are crooked, but she knows it not" (Proverbs 5:1–6).

"My son, keep your father's commands and do not forsake your mother's teaching. Bind them upon your heart forever; fasten them around your neck. When you walk, they will guide you; when you sleep they will watch over you; when you awake, they will speak to you. For these commands are a lamp, this teaching is a light, and the corrections of discipline are the way to life, keeping you from the immoral woman, from the smooth tongue of the wayward wife. Do not lust in your heart after her beauty or let her captivate you with her eyes, for the prostitute reduces you to a loaf of bread, and the adulteress preys upon your very life. Can a man scoop fire into his lap without his clothes being burned? Can a man walk on hot coals without his feet being scorched? So is he who sleeps with another man's wife; no one who touches her will go unpunished" (Proverbs 6:20–29).

See also Proverbs 7.

Jesus on Adultery

Our Lord often spoke out on this subject, raising its sinfulness from the physical act to the lustful thought. While he was quick to forgive repentant adulterers, He always condemned the practice as sin. Consider these statements:

"You have heard that it was said, 'Do not commit adultery.' But I tell you that anyone who looks at a woman lustfully has already committed adultery in his heart. If your right eye causes you to sin, gouge it out and throw it away. It is better for you to lose one part of your body than for your whole body to be thrown into hell. And if your right hand causes you to sin, cut it off and throw it away. It is better for you to lose one part of your body than for your whole body to go into hell.

"It has been said, 'Anyone who divorces his wife must give her a certificate of divorce.' But I tell you that anyone who divorces his wife, except for marital unfaithfulness, causes her to commit adultery, and anyone who marries a woman so divorced commits adultery" (Matthew 5:27–32).

"I tell you that anyone who divorces his wife, except for marital unfaithfulness, and marries another woman commits adultery" (Matthew 19:9).

"Now a man came up to Jesus and asked, 'Teacher, what good thing must I do to get eternal life?'

" 'Why do you ask me about what is good?' Jesus replied. 'There is only One who is good. If you want to enter life, obey the commandments.'

" 'Which ones?' the man inquired.

" Jesus replied, 'Do not murder, do not commit adultery, do not steal, do not give false testimony, honor your father and mother,' and 'love your neighbor as yourself' " (Matthew 19:16–19).

Other New Testament Passages

Adultery and fornication seem to be used interchangeably in some places in the New Testament. Fornication, which comes from the Greek word *porneia* literally means any sexual violation ranging from adultery to homosexuality, and it is always forbidden. The new Gentile converts from paganism were given the following mandate by the early church elders:

"It seemed good to the Holy Spirit and to us not to burden you with anything beyond the following requirements: You are to abstain from food sacrificed to idols, from blood, from the meat of strangled animals and from sexual immorality. You will do well to avoid these things" (Acts 15:28–29).

"Do you not know that the wicked will not inherit the kingdom of God? Do not be deceived: Neither the sexually immoral nor idolaters nor adulterers nor male prostitutes nor homosexual offenders nor thieves nor the greedy not drunkards nor slanderers nor swindlers will inherit the kingdom of God" (1 Corinthians 6:9–10).

"The body is not meant for sexual immorality, but for the Lord, and the Lord for the body. . . . Flee from sexual immorality. All other sins a man commits are outside his body, but he who sins sexually sins against his own body. Do you not know that your body is a temple of the Holy Spirit, who is in you, whom you have received from God? You are not your own" (1 Corinthians 6:13, 18–19).

"But among you there must not be even a hint of sexual immorality, or of any kind of impurity, or of greed, because these are improper for God's holy people. Nor should there be obscenity, foolish talk or coarse joking, which are out of place, but rather thanksgiving. For of this you can be sure: No immoral, impure or greedy person—such a man is an idolater—has any inheritance in the kingdom of Christ and of God" (Ephesians 5:3–5).

"Put to death, therefore, whatever belongs to your earthly nature: sexual immorality, impurity, lust, evil desires and greed, which is idolatry. Because of these, the wrath of God is coming" (Colossians 3:5–6).

"It is God's will that you should be holy; that you should

avoid sexual immorality; that each of you should learn to control his own body in a way that is holy and honorable, not in passionate lust like the heathen, who do not know God; and that in this matter no one should wrong his brother or take advantage of him. The Lord will punish men for all such sins, as we have already told you and warned you. For God did not call us to be impure, but to live a holy life. Therefore, he who rejects this instruction does not reject man but God, who gives you his Holy Spirit" (1 Thessalonians 4:3–8).

It is quite apparent from these verses that God's standard is unchanging and absolute. If we are to live holy lives, we must discipline and control our sexual drive, confining it to the one human relationship God allows— marriage. To the world, as expressed so loudly by the liberals who control much of our media, educational system, and entertainment industry, that is unthinkable. Because they often deny the existence of a personal holy God, they naturally deny moral absolutes. But the Scriptures reflect the mind of God, making it clear that whether three thousand years before Christ or in the twenty-first century, God's standards of morality are ever the same.

WHAT ABOUT PETTING?

We have already dealt with dating and petting, but in this scriptural context it should be pointed out that petting is a prelude to intercourse. In marriage we call it foreplay. The danger of petting is that it never satisfies but reflects a natural God-given quest for "more, more, more" until coitus culminates the sexual tensions of husband and wife. This is natural, beautiful, and meaningful.

However, because adultery is so consistently con- demned by God, wise parents will teach their teenagers that foreplay or petting (which may well be the most exciting activity they have ever engaged in) only leads to frustration or adultery. In obedience to God, petting must be avoided. It never fosters love on a lasting basis and, if engaged in long enough, will lead to adultery.

Few if any Christian young people deliberately decide to commit adultery. They usually become sexually intimate with those they love and eventually encounter irresistible temptation. For that reason it is best to conclude that since adultery is definitely wrong, those activities that lead to adultery are likewise wrong.

10

What Do We Do When Everything Goes Wrong?

"MY DAUGHTER IS pregnant and she is only seventeen!" cried a brokenhearted mother. "What should I do?"

"My son just got his girlfriend pregnant and they are both still in high school. What should we do?" mourned another parent.

These cries for help are real, and they are not uncommon. Almost every pastor has heard them many times. The fear of an unwed pregnancy is present with many parents. There were one million teenage unwed pregnant girls in America last year, which means there were two million families thrust into heartache and crisis.

One of the first reactions of parents is to place blame. "Where did we go wrong?" or "Why did the church fail us?" The truth is, it does little good to waste time fixing blame. Indeed, a parent can do everything right and still be faced with moral tragedy.

PREVENTING PREGNANCY OUT OF WEDLOCK

There is no foolproof way for parents to prevent a teen pregnancy, for everything still depends on our children's exercise of their free will. No one can watch over his teen twenty-four hours a day. However, the percentage of teen pregnancies is much lower in homes with sex education than in the average household. Here are some qualities that in my opinion will help teens resist promiscuity and avoid unwanted pregnancies:

- A warm, loving relationship between parents;
- Strong religious beliefs that are practiced in the home;
- Sex education in the home that treats sexuality as normal and beautiful and provides an easy communication on the subject between children and parents;
- Thorough instruction in moral values based on the Word of God that makes God's standards clear;
- A consistent avoidance of sexually debasing TV programs, movies, magazines, or conversation in or out of the home;
- Close surveillance of a teen's friends that prohibits fellowship with those who do not share the values of the home;
- Fairly rigid adherence to rules for dating;
- Active participation in church and Christian youth activities;
- Exaltation of morality and virtue in marriage;
- A consistent teaching of responsibility in all of life;
- An abundance of parental prayer.

Following these guidelines will reduce the likelihood of our teens' becoming sexually active. But remember that they are not foolproof.

"IT'S THE NICE GIRLS WHO GET PREGNANT"

A disconsolate father of four children called and identified himself as a supporter of our ministry, a medical doctor, and an active member of his church. Then he said, "My oldest daughter will be seventeen next month and she is pregnant. She is a straight-*A* student with only one year of high school left. Would it be possible for you to let her come to San Diego and attend your Christian high school? I will be happy to pay for her board and room with a Christian family."

Then the man said something I have heard many times: "My daughter said she got pregnant the first and only time she ever had sex. I believe her." I told her father that it is usually the nice girls who get pregnant. Naughty girls on dates take steps to avoid pregnancy.

This Christian girl had made a dreadful mistake that was entirely out of character for her. In spite of how it sounds, she was a very spiritual girl with a sincere desire to serve the Lord. Her loving, supportive parents testified, "She has never been a rebellious daughter and has never given us a moment of trouble before." Fortunately, she repented of her sin, really sought God's direction in her life, and today is a well-adjusted Christian wife and mother.

We might ask, "How could that happen?" The answer is, very gradually. This fine Christian girl committed a sin of passion that almost ruined her life. Like thousands of other teenagers, she and her "steady" boyfriend began making out one night when she just happened to be most fertile in her monthly cycle. At that time a young woman's emotions are highly combustible. Her emotions got out of control and she did what she never dreamed she would ever do. Kissing led to petting, petting led to intercourse, and she came home feeling very guilty. Then she found out she was pregnant.

Could this ever happen to your daughter? Given the right circumstances, any Christian is vulnerable to any sin, if he or she makes the first compromise. That is why the Bible teaches that playing with sin is extremely dangerous. We should avoid sin rather than trying to get as close to it as possible without getting burned. People who take the risks usually get burned.

It was this unfortunate girl's lot to commit a sin that carries with it the heaviest consequences. In her case it was "8 pounds 7 ounces" and much heartache for her and every member of her family. The girl stayed in her parents' home until she was four months along. By that time she could no longer keep her condition secret from her younger sisters and brothers and her friends, so she came to San Diego to live with a Christian family in our church. We could not admit her to our high school, but we arranged private tutoring so she could finish her eleventh year in time to return home and graduate with her class after the birth of her child.

WHAT SHOULD A PARENT DO?

I have counseled many Christian families through teenage pregnancies and have made some observations on how to handle the situation. First and foremost, face the problem head-on without recriminations and accusations. "How could you do such a thing?" is no way to greet a daughter when she makes her tragic announcement. If ever she needed love and acceptance, it is at that moment. She is terrified and guilt-stricken enough. She needs to know that God forgives her (if she has repented), and she needs her parents' forgiveness. It may be difficult for her to understand and accept God's forgiveness if she does not receive forgiveness from her parents.

One of the saddest cases I have dealt with concerned an eighteen-year-old girl in the youth group of our church during the early days of our ministry. The girl's father was so angry and humiliated that he kicked her out of the house and never let her return. She became angry and rebellious toward her father and toward God. The situation eventually destroyed her parents' marriage.

True love is unconditional. At a time like this, a girl needs to know that, like the Prodigal Son, she is continually loved by her parents. We love our children because they are our children, not because they do everything right. The important thing for parents at this point is to show that although this was her sin, they will help her through this trial.

As tragic as it is, this is not the end of her life. Thousands of young women have risen above this kind of crisis to live effective and useful lives. But this is much easier to achieve when she has loving, supportive parents.

SHOULD SHE MARRY THE FATHER?

Should a pregnant girl marry the father of her unborn child? In some cases she should. But not in every instance. If the father is unsaved, she definitely should not marry him. That would violate Scripture (2 Corinthians 6:12) and may well sentence her to a lifetime of marital misery. If the couple are both Christians and had been engaged or were talking about marriage, and if both parents concur, it may be wise to speed up their wedding plans.

Most of the time, however, a decision to marry because of pregnancy means only following one giant mistake with an even bigger one. The divorce rate is catastrophic among young people who decided to marry due to pregnancy. Marriage interferes with their educational and vocational potential. It usually thrusts the young man into the market-place without adequate skills or the opportunity to develop them; it forces him to try to support a family on minimum wages that will barely sustain one life. Such a couple have two strikes against them before they even begin to live as a family.

It is far better for the couple to deal with the consequences of the unplanned pregnancy as best they can and seek as much as possible to resume normal lives. Although pregnancy without marriage is a tragedy for all concerned, it is not the end of the world. Placing the responsibilities of marriage and parenting on teenagers is rarely the best solution.

WHAT ABOUT THE FATHER?

Women seem to bear the greatest consequences of teenage promiscuity and unplanned pregnancy. Occasionally I have counseled young women who were so promiscuous that they did not know who had fathered their child. That is not usually the case. Most girls have no problem identifying the father of their child. So what about the father? It is very important that he not abdicate his responsibility for this new life.

I recommend that the father of the girl arrange a meeting with all the people concerned—the two young people and their parents. At that meeting the parents of the boy need to be confronted with his sin. Not in a judgmental way, like the Pharisees who wanted to stone only the woman taken in adultery, for obviously two people are involved in the sin. But his parents must know what he has done; if he is a minor, they are responsible for him.

The father needs first of all to recognize his actions as sinful and repent of them. Shame often encourages repentance and turning to the Lord. If the father is saved, this should cause him to turn back to Christ; if he is unsaved, he needs to accept the Savior. He and his parents also need to acknowledge his lack of moral standards. If properly counseled, this young man can become motivated to live a productive life with a new respect for the sanctity of sex and the importance of self-control. If he rejects the offers to repent, he is likely to continue to misuse his sexuality.

IS ABORTION AN OPTION?

One question that is bound to surface is, What about an abortion? The standard argument for those who allow abortion is that it can be performed legally and safely in a hospital. In one month's time the whole crisis of a pregnancy out of wedlock would be over.

The problem is, two wrongs never make a right. Abortion may be legal, but it shouldn't be. Regardless of what the justices of the U.S. Supreme Court decided in 1973, abortion is murder. It is not an option for a Christian family.

A couple dealing with pregnancy desperately need the blessing and guidance of God at this time. The last thing they should do is add murder to adultery. Besides, the crisis wouldn't be over in a month. Abortion advocates don't warn women that post-abortion depression is very common. I have conducted the funeral services of some women who committed suicide after having abortions. Moreover, women who have had abortions tend to have more difficulty sustaining a pregnancy later on; some have to forego motherhood altogether. Many women carry their guilt to the grave. As difficult as it is to carry an unwanted pregnancy to full term, it is far better than suffering the weight of abortion guilt for a lifetime.

At the first Washington conference of Concerned Women for America, my wife Beverly, the president of CWA, presented a graphic pro-life film message that showed an actual abortion. Before the showing to the twenty-one hundred women was completed, twenty-seven of them left the room, weeping. One fled screaming, "They lied to me! They didn't tell me it was like that!" All twenty-seven of these women had had abortions, some of them many years before; none of them could handle the guilt of knowing they had killed another human being. Only by asking God's forgiveness through His Son's death on the cross is there cleansing for their sin and peace with God (see 1 John 1:7, 9).

WHO SHOULD PAY?

It is my view that the boy and his parents should pay *all* the medical and preliminary expenses of his child. This should include the cost of prenatal care, hospital delivery and doctor's fees, board and room for the girl if she goes to another city to have the child, and travel costs. The total costs may reach $2,500 or more, but I consider it imperative that the young man assume responsibility for them.

A girl pays a price in nine months of carrying the child, of shame, pain, and estrangement from her family, and in postnatal care. The least the boy should pay are the expenses. He may have to borrow the money from his parents until he can earn it. It will do him no good to avoid his responsibility by ignoring the girl's plight or by letting his parents bear the financial consequences of his actions. Either way, he loses—his material well-being or some of his manhood.

It might take a young man eight-to-nine hundred hours of work at minimum wages to defray the expenses, but it will help him to grow up if he is forced to take full responsibility for what he has done.

If he and his parents refuse to bear this responsibility, the girls' parents have two options. If he is unsaved and refuses, they should hire a good attorney and force him to bear the expenses. If the boy's family are Christians and refuse, then they should be taken before the church. A group of church leaders of his congregation and the girl's church (if they attend different churches) should sit in counsel and make a binding declaration. It is not in the boy's best interest to avoid financial responsibility in this matter.

SHOULD SHE ADOPT OUT OR KEEP THE CHILD?

The big question that my broken-hearted doctor friend had to face was, Should my daughter offer the baby for adoption by a Christian couple, or should she raise the child herself? Since I first began counseling people in this kind of situation, there has been a complete reversal in social practice. Thirty years ago a single woman almost never kept her child. Today most of them do. A recent survey indicated that 90 percent of unwed mothers keep their children.

My counsel has always been the same, and even though it is seldom followed, I still believe it is right. The mother-to-be should decide what is best for her child and do it. The current custom of girls' keeping their babies is, in my opinion, based on self-interest, not on the child's best interest.

A young actress appeared on a network TV talk show to discuss her pregnancy. A leading teenage idol, she was asked, "Are you going to marry your live-in boyfriend now that you're expecting?"

"Oh, my no!" she replied. "We aren't ready for marriage yet."

She was asked, "Do you intend to keep your baby?"

"Oh, yes! I can't wait to have this baby. In fact, I want several babies."

The talk-show hostess couldn't hide her surprise and blurted, "Out of wedlock?"

And the starlet said, "Certainly. I may want them from different men."

As bizarre as that idea may seem, it is not totally just a fad. I have met an unmarried nurse who had three by design—each from a different man. She chose men whose mental and physical characteristics she admired, then seduced them. Thus she accrued "all the advantages of motherhood without the restrictions of having a husband."

These and other reports lead me to believe that we will be seeing a wave of deliberate pregnancies among unwed teenagers. It may be the next trend in the sexual revolution. We have seen unbelievable changes in our culture's moral code in the past three decades. It used to be a badge of shame for an unwed woman to raise a child alone; today it seems to be a badge of honor that is increasingly revered. One hopes this fad will not catch on among Christian young people.

In the case of the doctor's daughter, I urged that she do her best to keep her local friends from knowing anything about her condition, that she have her baby miles away from home, and that she let us help her find a Christian couple who could not have children of their own and would seek adoption. When she asked, "Why shouldn't I keep my baby?" I offered the following reasons:

1. Ideally, every child needs two Christian parents to love him and give him a balanced home, training, and example so that when the time comes for the youngster to marry and raise a family, he will have been exposed to a biblical role model. God will provide for the widow or unwillingly divorced mother who is left to raise children alone; but I am not certain He will make up the difference when a young woman deliberately chooses that lifestyle.

2. An unwed mother will probably have a difficult time providing even the basic essentials of life for her baby. In all probability, she will not be able to support her child's needs for a higher education and adequate training to reach his potential. Her decision could seriously limit the vocational potential of her child.

3. It is unlikely that the child will have the advantage of being raised with a brother or sister because his mother's opportunities for finding a Christian husband are sharply reduced. I know of several happy cases where a Christian man has married a single mother and adopted her child. But this is the exception, not the rule. Usually her motherhood would be a hindrance to her meeting and getting to know eligible men so that a love relationship could develop.

4. Motherhood will probably limit a single woman's finding "the perfect will of God" for her life. Placing the child for adoption has traditionally served the best interests of the baby and provided a means for the mother to pick up the pieces of her life, resume her education, and prepare herself as "a vessel unto honor fit for the master's use" (2 Timothy 2:21). In the long run, it is usually best for the advancement of the kingdom of God, in God's use of both lives, to place the child for adoption.

5. Most of a woman's reasons for keeping the child are selfish. Many unwed mothers who kept their children have told me, "I need someone to love." Many young women grow up today starved for love and turn to their children to fill that

need. This kind of love can lead to a "smother-mother" love that has a harmful effect on a child's psychological development.

6. Probably the hardest thing for a mother to do is to place her child for adoption. But when all the facts are considered, most Christian young women decide that it is best course of action. It is certainly better for a woman to go into her marriageable years unencumbered by children. Her life will go on, and her natural yearnings to share her life with someone else will grow. Besides, in a real sense, all parents raise their children for someone else. For a mother to decide to keep her child when she is age sixteen or seventeen may someday prove to be costly, even if she has the best of intentions; she may find herself alone again while she is still in her late thirties.

I offer one word of caution: In the case of unwed mothers we should make sure the children are adopted into Christian families that will raise them with the same spiritual values we hold. Once assured of that, we can commit the children to God and get on with the rest of life—which may last another sixty or seventy years.

My doctor friend's daughter took that advice. We found her son a fine Christian home, and she enrolled in a Christian college. Giving her son up for adoption was a heartrending decision for this young mother to make; but she made the right decision, and most of the time she knows it down deep in her heart.

SHOULD SHE TELL HER PROSPECTIVE HUSBAND?

If a single mother who adopts out her child eventually marries, she will face the question, Should I tell my prospective husband about my past? There is no universal answer to that question. Some young men are mature enough to handle that knowledge and some are not. If the woman has successfully kept her experience secret and there is little likelihood it will ever be revealed, it is probably best not to tell him. But usually this is not the case. Sometimes there is a person who could inadvertently let the truth slip out.

For this reason I usually suggest that the woman tell her suitor the truth—but only after he asks for her hand in marriage. She should *not* reveal it to just any man with whom she gets serious. If a Christian man falls in love with her, she owes him the truth rather than take a chance that her past will be revealed as a tragic surprise after marriage. Indeed, this disclosure can be a good test of how much he truly loves her. He will feel disappointed and disillusioned when she first tells him, but if he really loves her, he will realize that she is not the same person now as when she was a teenager. By God's grace he needs to see her as the godly woman she has become. If he rejects her because of this knowledge, she can reasonably conclude that his legalistic rigidity would have made him difficult to live with anyway.

This brings us to another important matter: guilt. Guilt seriously weakens self-esteem. This is particularly true in cases where a Christian woman has made the mistake of having sex out of wedlock. This sin, like any other, can be forgiven, of course. But two conditions accentuate this kind of guilt: (1) The church's standards of virtue and morality; and (2) the highly public aspect of pregnancy. We have indicated a way for unwed girls to maintain secrecy during pregnancy, but this is difficult to guarantee.

For these and other reasons, a Christian unwed mother is likely to have a difficult time regaining her self-respect and rebuilding a strong self-image. This is partly because she is confronted with the fact of her sin every day for at least nine months. By the time her baby is born, her self-image is usually devastated. That is one reason why her family should never condemn her once she has acknowledged her sin and received God's forgiveness. She needs their reassurance and encouragement to realize that in our day it is wrong to assume that dropping one's guard and making the youthful mistake of engaging in premarital sex does not indicate a permanent character flaw. Who of us as adults would like to be judged on the basis of our behavior as teenagers?

Many young people have let God use the experience of parenthood out of wedlock to prove their dependence on Him for grace and power to become godly adults. This tragic experience is not the end of a person's life. With God's help and adherence to His principles for living, they can become strong in the Lord and in the power of His might.

CHANGE THEIR DATING POLICY

After the whole matter of unwed parenthood is dealt with as suggested, one more thing must be considered: prevention against recurrence. This experience should teach both the boy and the girl about the weakness of the flesh and the high cost of sin. Such a lesson should warn them and their parents that new standards of behavior must be followed. The dating rules prescribed in this book should be followed carefully, and neither person should ever again let himself or herself get physically involved with the opposite sex before marriage. True love never requires sex in order to develop. Lust demands sex. As we have explained, a relationship built on physical attraction will cloud the other attributes and confuse even the most mature judgment. Sin is always avoided best by reducing the opportunities for temptation.

A BEAUTIFUL STORY

As a woman spoke to me between sessions at a Family Life Seminar in Virginia Beach, Virginia, I had the feeling that I had seen her before, but she assured me that we had never met. Then she asked if I recalled a handsome young man from my former pastorate in San Diego. Yes, I did. I even remembered when he was a baby and had watched him grow to be a fine young man. I expected that one day he might go into the ministry.

The woman shocked me by saying, "I am his mother!"

"How could that be?" I asked. I knew his parents well, for they were active members in my congregation. But as I looked into her face I noticed that it was almost like looking at the youth she claimed was her son.

Then she told me her story. When she was a young, single girl, she got pregnant and placed her son for adoption Later she married and had three other children, but she never forgot her son. About fifteen years after the adoption took place, she received Christ and was totally transformed. A year later her husband was saved. One night she had a dream that so disturbed her, both she and her husband woke up. She was so distraught, her husband urged her to talk about it. So she told him about her teenage pregnancy and confessed her great concern that her son become a Christian.

At the urging of her understanding and loving husband, she began a vigorous search for her son and somehow traced him to San Diego. Imagine how thrilled she was to discover that in the providence of God her son had been adopted by Christian parents and had known Christ longer than she did! Since their reunion the young man has spent half of one summer getting acquainted with his natural mother; both sets of parents are becoming good friends, though they live three thousand miles apart.

All parents of unwed mothers, as well as the mothers themselves, should remember one principle when contemplating placing their children for adoption to Christian parents: Jesus said, "Suffer the little children to come unto me, for of such is the Kingdom of God." He is more interested in bringing them to Himself than we are.

11

Venereal Disease

A GRAVE CONSEQUENCE of America's sexual revolution is the ever-increasing problem of venereal disease infecting large numbers of people. It is estimated that as many as 21 million Americans now suffer from incurable genital herpes (Herpes Simplex II); approximately one million men and women contract gonorrhea each year; and more than 100,000 cases of syphilis are recorded annually. These are the *reported* cases. In addition, we are now facing one of the most serious threats of all, the AIDS epidemic— first identified in the homosexual community, among intravenous drug users, and among Haitian refugees. The disease is now spreading into the heterosexual community, especially through contaminated blood transfusions.

According to King Holmes, former president of the American Venereal Disease Association, "There are twenty or more genital infections known to be spread by sexual intercourse, and the incidence of several has been increasing at epidemic rates during the last decade."[1] The most dangerous, of course, are gonorrhea, syphilis, genital herpes, and AIDS. Other forms of VD include trichomoniasis, nongonococcal urethritis, monilia, crabs, and scabies.

GONORRHEA

One of the most common slang terms for gonorrhea is "the clap." The gonococcus germ that causes this disease incubates in two to ten days, causing painful urination and a discharge of pus from the penis. In "asymptomatic gonorrhea" there are no symptoms in males. This means that an infected man can unknowingly transmit the disease to others.

Women commonly reflect no visible symptom of gonorrhea, which makes the disease very dangerous. When a woman is infected, the gonococcus germs multiply around the cervix, causing a thick pus discharge. In addition, they often move up into the Fallopian tubes, which can cause pelvic inflammatory disease (PID). This can be treated, but scar tissue may block the Fallopian tubes, causing sterility. If the tubes are only partially blocked, there is also danger of tubal pregnancies. Gonorrhea poses a risk to unborn babies. If the mother has contracted gonorrhea, the baby can be infected as it passes through the birth canal. A baby's eyes are particularly vulnerable. Once infected, blindness often results. Doctors now routinely put silver nitrate drops or penicillin ointments in a newborn's eyes to avoid venereal infection. Nevertheless, a baby can be infected at birth through his nose, mouth, or rectum.

Gonorrhea can cause inflammation of the testicle in men and sterility, arthritis, and heart disease in both men and women.

SYPHILIS

This disease is caused by spirochetes, which multiply rapidly in the body and attack normal tissues—especially the bones, joints, liver, heart, large blood vessels, eyes, spinal cord, and brain. Four stages characterize the disease. In the primary stage, the person develops a "chancre" or sore, either on his lips, inside his mouth, or on the genitals. In the second stage, he develops a rash and loses hair. In the third stage, called the "latent period," no symptoms are visible and a person can unknowingly pass the disease on to others. During the "late" stage, a person may suffer heart disease, brain damage, paralysis, and blindness.

HERPES SIMPLEX II

Twenty-one million Americans (nearly 10 percent of the population) now suffer from the incurable venereal disease Herpes Simplex II. During the first week after infection, clusters of blisters develop on the penis, labia, thighs, lower abdomen, buttocks, and anus. These blisters often break, causing excruciating pain. The person with herpes also experiences tenderness in the groin, a sick stomach, and fever. In June 1984, researchers announced they had discovered a possible treatment (not a cure) for herpes called Acyclovir (trade name: Zovirax). This medicine will help to relieve the pain caused by blisters.

NONGONOCOCCAL URETHRITIS

Nongonococcal urethritis or NGU, is caused by a strain of bacteria known as *Chlamydia trachomatia*. These bacteria incubate after about five days and infect the urethra, causing painful urination. This form of VD reflects the same general symptoms as gonorrhea. There are an estimated four to nine million new cases each year.

TRICHOMONIASIS

Trichomoniasis is caused by protozoa called *Trichomonas vaginalis*. It incubates after four-to-twenty days, usually in seven days. In women it produces a vaginal itch, pain in the pelvic area, and a yellowish-green discharge. Men seldom reflect any symptoms, though some experience itching and a whitish discharge from the penis in the morning, or less commonly in the evening.

MONILIA

The fungus of Monilia, or yeast, is often present in the female genital tract and bowels. The infection produces swelling, redness, a burning sensation in the genitals, and a whitish discharge.

CRABS

The term "crabs" refers to a body louse, *Pthirus pubis,* which creates an itching sensation when it bites.

SCABIES

The tiny mite, *Sarcopes scabiei,* causes redness and an itchy rash. Linear burrows can be seen on the person's body.

These are the major forms of VD with the exception of AIDS. In reviewing some of the literature available on such diseases, I was fascinated by the rationalizations of those writing the material. The American consensus is illustrated by a comment made by Eric Johnson in his book, *V.D.*:

> A major enemy in the war against VD is *do nothing*; a fancier word for it is *apathy.* Two other enemies are the embarrassment and guilt that arise when people confuse *moral* questions and *health* questions. Of course, if sexual intercourse were limited to married couples who were faithful to each other, the problem of VD would be much easier to solve—but, whether we like it or not, there is no such limit on intercourse and other sexual contact.[2]

In my opinion, Johnson is misguided. VD is definitely a health problem, but it represents a very serious moral problem as well, for it is a direct result of men and women throwing aside traditional morality. Another fact sheet reads, "Aside from abstinence, the only means of preventing the spread of VD during intercourse is for a man to wear a condom, called a 'safe' or 'rubber,' available at any drugstore." Both Johnson and the writer of the fact sheet know the real solution to the VD problem: total abstinence from sexual intercourse until marriage, and then faithfulness to the marriage partner. That kind of moral behavior is absolutely essential for anyone who calls himself a Christian.

Your teenagers or young adults need never fear any form of venereal disease if they obey the Word of God concerning sexual conduct. Only those who are sexually promiscuous and immoral risk getting VD and causing harm to many other people by spreading the disease through sexual intercourse. I wonder how many unfaithful husbands have given their wives incurable herpes? Or how many unfaithful women have infected their unborn babies with venereal disease? My counseling experience suggests that there are far more than most people realize.

The spread of venereal disease in our society is the penalty for discarding God's clear teachings on sexual matters. Perhaps the most frightening form of VD is AIDS, which is reaching out to destroy not only the sexually promiscuous—but the innocent as well.

AIDS

Dr. James Curran, head of the AIDS task force at the Centers for Disease Control in Atlanta, recently made this sobering comment: "It's not just a 'gay' disease. It is spreading fast and all of us can get it. At this point we can't say when it will end. We have no cure. I think thousands more people will die of this disease before it's over."[3] Mervyn Silverman, former head of San Francisco's health department, has called AIDS "the most devastating epidemic of the century."[4]

AIDS (Acquired Immune Deficiency Syndrome) is a

disease believed to be caused by a virus, HTLV-III, that attacks the body's immune system, destroying the ability of the body to fight off sickness. When this happens, any simple problem can quickly become a life or death matter. Many AIDS victims die from pneumonia or develop rare forms of cancer.

The disease first appeared in the homosexual community but since then has been traced to Haitian refugees and intravenous drug users. Medical science has found no cure, and thus AIDS inevitably kills its victims. As of December 1984, researchers identified 7,270 victims and 3,449 deaths. By mid-1985 health officials were reporting that fullly 50 percent of the known AIDS victims had died. Studies also indicated that as many as 300,000 other people have been exposed to the AIDS virus; of those, approximately 10 percent will eventually get AIDS.

How does a person contract the disease? Homosexuals get it through intimate contact—the exchange of blood and semen during anal intercourse or oral sex. Drug users get it through contaminated needles, and innocent victims are now being subjected to it through blood transfusions. If an AIDS victim donates blood at a hospital or through a Red Cross outlet, he is infecting that blood supply with deadly disease.

Hemophiliacs suffer because of the AIDS epidemic. In October 1984, the American Red Cross had to recall nineteen hundred bottles of blood clotting agent used by hemophiliacs. The reason? An AIDS victim had donated plasma at a Red Cross center.

AIDS has claimed the lives of innocent people. In September 1983, a newborn baby at a Boston hospital died after receiving a contaminated blood transfusion; in December 1984, a medical technician in Boston contracted the disease when he accidentally pricked himself with an AIDS-contaminated needle. In April 1984, a patient at the West Virginia University Hospital died after having an AIDS-contaminated blood transfusion.

This disease is not confined to the homosexual community or to drug users, but is spreading rapidly among heterosexual people who are promiscuous. Dr. Anthony Fauci, director of the National Institute of Allergy and Infectious Diseases in Bethesda, Maryland, had noted, "It may not be too long before promiscuous heterosexual men and women become another high-risk group."[5]

AIDS is threatening to kill thousands of innocent people because immoral people chose to have perverted sex. What is the attitude of the homosexual population? According to an article in *Time* magazine, homosexuals are more concerned about finding a cure for AIDS than changing their lifestyles. The article contained a photograph of men sitting in a "gay" bar. On the counter is a sign warning them about AIDS. It read, "AIDS is everyone's problem. Protect yourself and those you love. Use condoms. Avoid any exchange of body fluids. Limit your use of recreational drugs. Enjoy more time with fewer partners. AIDS is not spread through casual contact."[6]

In May 1983, Robert Schwab, an AIDS victim and homosexual activist in Texas, observed, "If it takes threatening, and perhaps giving blood to get us the money, the research funds we need, that may be it. That doesn't mean I'm condoning that. . . . I think as long as gay people are dying in droves . . . I think whatever action is required to get national attention is valid. If that includes blood terrorism, so be it."[7]

Are homosexuals actually waging blood terrorism against an innocent populace to obtain freedom from the fear of death? Who knows? I believe, that America is facing one of the most serious epidemics in history. Hemophiliacs, babies, medical technicians, and all the rest of us now run the risk of contracting an incurable venereal disease through contaminated blood transfusions. Only God knows where this new epidemic will end. But unless medical science finds a cure or unless our nation's sexual habits change, this disease could take the lives of half of this nation's population by the year 2000.

A nurse I know came within an eyelash of contracting AIDS. While drawing blood from a patient *suspected* of having AIDS, the patient thrashed about, and the needle came out and stabbed my friend's hand—one of the known ways of transmitting the disease. Fortunately for the nurse, the patient's report turned up negative. If he had been an AIDS victim, my innocent friend would have faced a 50 percent chance of dying.

If very many people in the medical field were to die as innocent victims of this disease, there would be an outcry of national proportions. It would be tragic to wait until "enough" people have died before our society decides to take action against the conditions that allow this disease to spread. It is amazing to me that everyone doesn't see that our country is desperately in need of moral and spiritual revival.

What Every Parent Needs to Know About Sex

in Case His Children Should Ask

THIS BOOK WOULD not be complete without an alphabetical list of categories covering every imaginable subject parents will be confronted with by inquisitive children. When children ask their endless stream of questions, it is a healthy sign to us as parents. It means we have a good relationship with them and can be their teachers instead of someone else who doesn't share our values.

Whenever a child or teenager asks a question you don't know the answer to, don't panic. Just look him in the eye and say, "I'm not sure myself. Give me some time and I'll find an answer." Or you might say, "Let's look that up in this family book."

No one knows all the answers on the subject of sex, so we need never feel threatened if we come up blank. However, there is good material available today in Christian bookstores. If you don't find the answer under one of the following headings, please consult the bibliography in this book, or my book *The Act of Marriage,* or Dr. Ed Wheat's book, *Intended for Pleasure** (particularly for people who are contemplating marriage).

ABORTION

There is no more emotionally explosive issue in the United States and Canada today than abortion. Five decades of the teaching of evolution in our schools had created such a low view of human life that abortion came to be considered largely just a therapeutic treatment of no consequence. After all, if humans are just animals, then an unborn fetus is a living mass without personhood. The Supreme Court reflected this view in 1973 when it voted seven to two in favor of legalizing abortion. Justice Harry Blackmun, writing the majority opinion said, "In short, the unborn have never been recognized in the law as persons in the whole sense." Since then, more than 17 million babies have been murdered in the name of abortion. While some would have us believe these abortions were therapeutic necessities, the truth is that most of them were performed out of the selfish motives of the mother.

U.S. Sen. Orrin Hatch wrote that medical research has established that "only 3 percent of all abortions are performed for therapeutic reasons or due to rape." This would mean that 97 percent of all abortions performed now are nothing but cold-blooded murder. Although lethargic on this issue for most of the seventies, the Christian community has finally found courage to join with Roman Catholics and pro-life groups to exercise political leverage. It is difficult at this time for any candidate to get elected to federal office who does not oppose federal funding for abortions. I predict that sentiment will grow until some kind of legislation is passed that will protect the life of the unborn. If the matter were put

---

*Old Tappan, N.J.: Fleming H. Revell, 1981.

to a vote of the people today, I believe it would be enacted into law, particularly after the third trimester or thirteenth week of pregnancy. As we noted earlier, the fetus is a complete human being after the third month. When people understand that, they overwhelmingly oppose abortion.

Medically speaking, "abortion" refers to the ending of a pregnancy before the fertilized egg or embryo or fetus has developed sufficiently to survive by itself outside the mother's womb. There are two kinds of abortion, "spontaneous" abortion (or "miscarriage," as it is commonly called) and "induced" abortion (when the fetus is deliberately or artificially removed.)

Not all miscarriages can be explained. Some women seem to have a difficult time sustaining a pregnancy, particularly during the first trimester. In some cases it seems to be nature's way of eliminating a life with potential birth defects. A miscarriage is an act of God and should not leave the mother with a sense of guilt over the death of her child.

Induced abortion is quite another matter. It is performed deliberately by forcibly extracting the fetus from the uterus of the mother. In some cases this is done by suction, in others by forceps. The cervix is stretched and the embryo is drawn out through the vagina after scraping the uterine walls with a knife called a "curette." This kind of surgery is often called a "D and C" (dilation and curettage).

I have seen pictures of some "surgical techniques" that showed the doctor actually pulling the baby's body parts out of the mother's womb in pieces. Although it sounds grotesque, it is true nevertheless that such abortions are an inhumane procedure that inflicts real torture upon an unborn child.

President Ronald Reagan was ridiculed by some pro-abortionists prior to his reelection campaign in early 1984 for citing medical research indicating that the unborn are capable of experiencing pain during an abortion. Later his critics were silenced by irrefutable medical evidence that supported his report. I have seen movies of a fluoroscope that shows a four-month-old-fetus shrinking away in pain in response to a metal probe that came close to its head—the same way any other normal human being would react. I also saw unmistakable evidence of pain on the face of the fetus just before his death by abortion. This may seem repulsive to some, but as Mrs. Dee Jepsen, former Special Assistant to the President, told the 1984 convention of the Concerned Women for America, "All we can lose is our lunch—the unborn lose their lives!"

There is no question that abortion is murder and should not be considered as an option by a Christian family. Admittedly, nine months of pregnancy and an unwed mother present many problems and heartaches for any Christian family. But they are not nearly so serious as carrying the burden of murder. I have known cases where authoritarian Christian parents insisted that their teenagers have abortions and came to regret it. They destroyed their testimony and moral credibility in the eyes of the most important people in those situations—their pregnant daughters. By contrast, I have seen several families trust God and stand up with their teens in that hour of crisis and have it change the course of their lives.

As stated earlier, pro-choice advocates don't mention the guilt women often carry after an abortion. Dr. Grace Ketterman, a psychiatrist, told about her work as the director of a maternity home where more than nine hundred pregnant young women came under her care and how the Supreme Court's decision in 1973 made abortion as a promising means of instantly solving their problems. She said, however, that after some time, "I began to be consulted by a pitiful parade of girls needing help. They had had abortions; sometimes more than one. They were full of remorse for their irresponsible taking of human life—unborn to be sure, but life nevertheless."[1]

I wonder how much the high suicide rate among teenagers today is affected by depression caused by the guilt that follows abortion.

Another harmful effect of abortion is that it can cause sterility or make it extremely difficult for a woman to sustain a pregnancy. I have counseled several women who because of induced abortions could not have children later. Each one carried the weight of guilt in knowing that she could never hold a child of her own in her arms or present one to her husband, who likewise wanted to be a father.

The Bible teaches, "The way of transgressors is hard" (Proverbs 13:15 KJV). We do not resolve the sin of adultery by covering it up with the sin of murder without bringing additional judgment on ourselves. Our teens need to understand that God has always put a high priority on human life. The greatest object of His love is human beings, because it was for human beings that He sacrificed His only Son. If an unplanned pregnancy burdens your family, you will face a severe test of your convictions. Make sure you don't fail your teen in the moment of testing, for the latter end will be worse than the first.

One important passage of Scripture in this connection is Exodus 21:22–23:

> "If men who are fighting hit a pregnant woman and she gives birth prematurely but there is no serious injury, the offender must be fined whatever the woman's husband demands and the court allows. But if there is serious injury, you are to take life for life. . . ."

God gave these words to Moses to teach the children of Israel that an unborn child deserved the same protection granted any other living person. He commanded that if a pregnant woman lost her child prematurely because a man injured her, the man must be put to death the same as any other murderer. The obvious implication is that the unborn is regarded by God as a living person.

ADULTERY

God expressly forbids adultery in the Ten Commandments. Exodus 20:14 states, "You shall not commit adultery." In

Matthew 5:27–28 Jesus reaffirms this prohibition and extends it even to lustful thoughts. He said in the Sermon on the Mount, "You have heard that it was said, 'Do not commit adultery.' But I tell you that anyone who looks at a woman lustfully has already committed adultery with her in his heart." The words *adultery* and *fornication* are used interchangeably in the Old and New Testaments. Both terms refer to a person's having sexual intercourse with someone to whom he or she is not married. Fornication includes other sinful acts such as incest.

Sexual intercourse is to be reserved *only* for a man and woman who have been joined together in marriage. All other sexual intercourse is considered adultery or fornication in the eyes of God and is condemned as sin. The person who commits adultery or fornication is not only sinning against God; the apostle Paul teaches that such a person also sins against his own body.

In 1 Corinthians 6:15–18 Paul writes,

Do you not know that your bodies are members of Christ himself? Shall I then take the members of Christ and unite them with a prostitute? Never! Do you not know that he who unites himself with a prostitute is one with her in body? For it is said, "The two will become one flesh." But he who unites himself with the Lord is one with him in spirit. Flee from sexual immorality. All other sins a man commits are outside his body, but he who sins sexually sins against his own body.

All sexual sin begins in the mind and then becomes action. The man who commits adultery does not suddenly decide to have an affair. There is a time of incubation long before he finally betrays his wife. Lustful thoughts planted by dirty magazines and films; watching scantily clad women at the beach; reading sexually arousing novels—all these and more gradually lead a man into sexual sin. Paul says "flee" from any temptation to engage in immorality. The person who continues to leave himself open to sexually stimulating materials is eventually going to fall. Once the sexual desire is ignited, watching nude women at the movies or reading sex books simply inflames that desire.

BIRTH CONTROL

There are no specific references to birth control in Scripture, so in my opinion it is a morally neutral subject. I believe that Christians should seek to bear children, but I do not think that the obligations and responsibilities should be imposed on a wife by the husband without her consent. The decision to have children should be a joint agreement reached through discussion and prayer between the husband and wife. No woman should be expected to keep bearing children from marriage through menopause. I know one man who had fathered five children close together, several of whom were conceived against his wife's will. She was physically and emotionally exhausted from bearing these children—and I believe she had been treated unfairly by a selfish husband.

I am only in favor of birth-control methods that do not destroy a fertilized egg. The various methods of birth control include some that prevent sperm from reaching the egg and some that actually kill a fetus.

The Pill is the most popular and probably the most reliable artificial means of contraception. The pill controls ovulation by changing the hormonal balance in a woman's body; it prevents an egg from being released into the Fallopian tubes. It is probably the most reliable form of contraception on the market. When it was first marketed, there were reported side effects, but these problems have been minimized by additional development and the discovery that smaller, safer doses are just as effective in preventing conception. (It is unfortunate that this birth-control device has also been instrumental in "liberating" women from traditional morality. The Pill has made premarital sexual intercourse "safe"—though it is still immoral in God's sight.)

Anyone considering this method of birth control should be advised that many researchers believe the Pill can also work as an 'abortifacient' in creating an irritation on the uterine wall that causes a fertilized egg to be expelled. I have read varying views among experts. It seems that the weaker dosages of the Pill, while lessening unpleasant side effects, allow for conception but irritate the embryo and cause abortion. For that reason I no longer recommend the Pill as an acceptable means of birth control.

The Condom. This contraceptive device—also known as a "rubber," "prophylactic," "pro," or "sheath"—is the second-most popular form of birth control in the United States. The condom first came into use in the fifteenth century as a protection against syphilis. It is a rubbery device that fits tightly over the penis like a snug glove. During intercourse, the condom catches the ejaculated sperm, preventing it from entering the woman's vagina.

There are several advantages to the condom. It is available over the counter at drugstores. There are no side effects. It is easy to use and its effectiveness immediately obvious. It also places responsibility for birth control on the husband, not the wife.

There are certain drawbacks, however. The condom may reduce the physical sensation experienced by the husband and often the wife experiences discomfort when the condom is not properly lubricated. Some condoms are already lubricated for comfort. Condoms manufactured in the United States must meet rigid government standards. The British and Japanese supply most of the condoms used in the rest of the world.

Vaginal Foam and Spermicides. These forms of contraception have been used for nearly thirty years with positive results. Statistics indicate that an average of only about 76 pregnancies occur for every thousand women using foams and spermicides. Foams, creams, and synthetic gels are available as spermicides, that is, products that kill the sperm without harming delicate vaginal tissues. Foams come in various forms such as in aerosol cans with applicators or in capsules that melt in the vagina.

Women who use spermicides often risk pregnancies because they fail to carefully follow the directions provided. Some research suggests that women who use spermicides incorrectly and become pregnant run a higher risk of having deformed babies or miscarriages. Following the directions explicitly is the best protection against such tragedies.

Rhythm Method. An unreliable method of birth control is known as the rhythm method. This requires the husband and wife to abstain from intercourse during the days just after ovulation. There are two methods of estimating the time of ovulation. One is the "temperature method," in which the wife takes her temperature each morning before getting out of bed. She marks this on a chart. A slight drop in temperature followed by a substantial increase indicates that ovulation has occurred during the drop in temperature. This record-keeping must be followed for months until clear patterns of ovulation can be discerned.

The second technique is the "calendar method." This requires keeping a record of the wife's menstrual cycle for eight months to a year. A formula can be used with this record to estimate when she is ovulating. A woman with a regular twenty-eight-day menstrual cycle will usually ovulate on the fourteenth day. From about the eighteenth day, no egg present would be present to be fertilized. The days before the eleventh day may also be safe. The problem is that some women can ovulate on any day of the month, so this method can be confusing, frustrating, and misleading.

To generalize on the rhythm method, it may be said that we can be reasonably certain that no contraceptives are needed one week before a woman's period, during the period, or five days afterward.

Diaphragm. I have described the diaphragm method of birth control in my book *The Act of Marriage*. The diaphragm is a strong, lightweight rubber cap somewhat smaller than the palm of the hand. It was the first medically accepted contraceptive, developed over forty years ago. The thin rim of the diaphragm is made of a ring-shaped, rubber-covered metal spring. Because the spring is flexible, the whole diaphragm can be compressed and passed easily into the vagina. It is then released in the upper widening canal of the vagina, where it covers the cervix like a dome-shaped lid.

The distance from the back wall of the vagina to the public bones varies from woman to woman. For this reason, diaphragms are made in a variety of sizes. During a pelvic examination that offers no discomfort to the woman, the doctor must measure this distance in order to select the proper diaphragm. . . . As properly instructed by the physician, the diaphragm must be inserted prior to intercourse, preferably several hours before entrance. If the diaphragm fits properly, neither mate should be aware of its presence.

The diaphragm acts as a barrier or deflector, preventing sperm from entering the uterus, but to be effective, it must be covered on the side next to the cervix with a spermicidal jelly or cream made for this purpose. . . . The diaphragm is a well-established, proven method which affords many women the security of the physical barrier in addition to the spermicide. The diaphragm has no effect on future fertility.[2]

IUD. The intrauterine device is actually not a contraceptive, but rather an abortifacient. It does not prevent the fertilization of the egg; it prevents the implantation of the fertilized egg on the wall of the uterus. In other words, the IUD is actually destroying the human embryo. It is about 90 percent effective as a birth control method, but it is technically an abortion device, not a contraception.

The IUD has been around for more than twenty-five hundred years, having first been invented on a primitive level in the Middle East by Arab camel drivers. These men, often traveling for years in desert caravans, had trouble dealing with pregnant camels. The beasts were no use to the drivers, but they would refuse to drop out of the caravans. Someone thought of the idea of placing an apricot pit in the uterus of the female camels to prevent pregnancy. They didn't understand how the apricot pit worked, but it proved to be an effective birth control device.

Today the typical IUD is made of plastic in various sizes and shapes. Some contain copper or the female hormone progesterone, which is released into the woman's body. The IUD is a soft, flexible plastic coil or oddly shaped disc that a physician must insert through the cervical canal into the uterine cavity, using a tube about the size of a soda straw. A small thread hangs from the IUD through the cervix to enable it to be removed. If a woman desires to become pregnant, she must go to a physician to have it removed. Interestingly enough, doctors are not really certain how the IUD works. They think that this foreign object changes the lining of the uterus and prevents the implantation of the fertilized egg.

The IUD is reliable, but has several drawbacks. Some women experience cramps or vaginal bleeding or pelvic discomfort. Other women's bodies simply expel the IUD as a foreign substance. Another possible side effect is perforation of the uterus. Recent discoveries indicate that long wear may produce some other dangerous side effects. Because the IUD is an abortion device, I do not recommend its use.

Coitus Interruptus. One of the least effective forms of birth control is "coitus interruptus" (or the "withdrawal method"). For this a man withdraws his penis from the woman's vagina just as he is about to ejaculate. This method is notoriously ineffective because sperm often leave the penis in lubricating fluids *before* ejaculation. This method also interrupts the romantic lovemaking that should be taking place between husband and wife. Instead of feeling unrestrained in their lovemaking, both partners feel tension, worrying that sperm might escape. In reality there are probably very few people in the country who effectively practice this method of birth control over a long period of time.

Abstinence. Among unmarried men and women, abstinence is the only absolutely guaranteed way to prevent an unwanted pregnancy and the resultant shame and conflict. Christians who are unmarried *must* practice abstinence or chastity if they are to obey the clear teachings of Scripture on sexual relations.

Married men and women are encouraged in Scripture to have sexual intercourse. In 1 Corinthians 7:3–5 the apostle Paul says,

> The husband should fulfill his marital duty to his wife, and likewise the wife to her husband. The wife's body does not belong to her alone but also to her husband. In the same way, the husband's body does not belong to him alone but also to his wife. Do not deprive each other except by mutual consent and for a time, so that you may devote yourselves to prayer.

CIRCUMCISION

Every baby boy comes into the world with a fold of flesh hanging over the head of his penis. This is called "the foreskin." It is usually surgically removed by a doctor a few days after birth. The process of removing this foreskin is called "circumcision." In Old Testament times the Jewish people performed circumcision as a religious rite eight days after the boy was born. This was performed in obedience to the Lord's command to Abraham recorded in Genesis 17:10–14. God told Abraham,

> This is my covenant with you and your descendants after you, the covenant you are to keep: Every male among you shall be circumcised. You are to undergo circumcision, and it will be the sign of the covenant between me and you. For the generations to come every male among you who is eight days old must be circumcised, including those born in your household or bought with money from a foreigner—those who are not your offspring. Whether born in your household or bought with your money, they must be circumcised. My covenant in your flesh is to be an everlasting covenant. Any

uncircumcised male, who has not been circumcised in the flesh, will be cut off from his people; he has broken my covenant.

Circumcision was not an option to the ancient Hebrews. It was a specific command of God that had to be obeyed. An uncircumcised man was to be cut off from his people.

Under the new covenant, instituted by Jesus Christ, Christians are free from this commandment given to Abraham. Circumcision is still routinely performed, but now there is new spiritual significance to this Old Testament custom. In Colossians 2:9–12 Paul writes,

> For in Christ all the fullness of the Deity lives in bodily form, and you have been given fullness in Christ, who is the head over every power and authority. In him you were also circumcised, in the putting off of the sinful nature, not with a circumcision done by the hands of men but with the circumcision done by Christ, having been buried with him in baptism and raised with him through your faith in the power of God, who raised him from the dead.

To a Christian, it doesn't matter whether or not a man's penis is circumcised. What does matter is that the person's heart is circumcised by removing the old sin nature.

Paul and Barnabas faced problems in dealing with the issue of circumcision among the Gentile and Hebrew converts. The Jewish Christians still believed that circumcision was mandatory, but Paul argued about the Mosaic Law before the Jerusalem Council and convinced the leadership that the ceremonial laws had been superseded by the new covenant under Jesus Christ. In response, the Christian leadership wrote a letter to the Gentile believers and gave them these simple instructions: "It seemed good to the Holy Spirit and to us not to burden you with anything beyond the following requirements: You are to abstain from food sacrificed to idols, from blood, from the meat of strangled animals and from sexual immorality. You will do well to avoid these things" (Acts 15:28-29 NIV).

The physical act of circumcision is done for hygienic reasons. With the foreskin removed, it is easier to keep the penis clean from possible infections, inflammations, and glandular secretions that might cause physical problems. In more primitive areas of the world, circumcision is still a religious rite or a rite of passage, indicating that a young man has entered adulthood.

EJACULATION / ORGASM

When a man's penis is manipulated either through masturbation or through foreplay, it fills up with blood and becomes stiff and erect in preparation for sexual intercourse. A special mixture of secretions from the prostate gland, seminal vesicles, and testicles produces the semen that will carry the sperm to their destination.

In addition, the Cowper's gland secretes a fluid that flows through the urethra, neutralizing the acids in the urine and providing lubrication during sexual intercourse. At the same time, a valve automatically shuts off, preventing any urine from escaping the bladder. During intercourse, the friction caused by the inward and outward thrusts of the penis in the vagina build up sexual energy in the man until there is an explosion of sperm from the urethra. This is known as ejaculation. It occurs from friction during masturbation as well. In every ejaculation, the average male discharges about a half-million sperm cells. Yet it requires only one cell to fertilize an egg during intercourse; the rest are discarded. Ejaculation in the male is also called an orgasm.

In a woman, orgasm results from the clitoris and vulva being manipulated during foreplay. These external sexual organs undergo physical changes. The clitoris hardens and becomes more sensitive in much the same way as a man's penis becomes erect. As the clitoris is continually manipulated, the woman moves toward orgasm. The clitoris has been described as the "sexual trigger" of a woman. Sometimes a woman does not learn to experience orgasm through intercourse until she has once achieved orgasm through manipulation by her husband's fingers. While some women feel uncomfortable at the suggestion of manual manipulation, most Christian counselors agree that it is a legitimate part of lovemaking between a husband and wife.

EXTERNAL ORGASM

The external orgasm, or coitus interruptus (see **Birth Control**), is an unreliable and dissatisfying means of preventing conception. A man would need an extraordinary amount of self-discipline to withdraw from his wife just at the moment when his sexual passion is at its height. Intercourse is a time for mutual surrender to fully enjoy lovemaking, not a time for "self-discipline." Coitus interruptus is unreliable for reasons other than passion, however. When the Cowper's gland begins secreting its lubricating fluid through the urethra, sperm cells often accompany it *before* ejaculation. Therefore, it is possible for a wife to get pregnant even without ejaculation into her vagina.

FANTASY

To fantasize or to think about having sexual relations with someone you're not married to is a sin condemned in Scripture. In Matthew 5:28 Jesus speaks of the sin of adultery in terms that no one had heard before. He reaffirms the Old Testament teaching that it was sinful to commit the act of adultery, but He says that it is just as bad to *think* unchaste thoughts about another person. These evil thoughts or imaginations are what we call "fantasy" today. In Philippians 4:8 Paul discusses the importance of keeping our minds focused on the good and the true. He encourages the Philippian Christians, "Finally, brothers, whatever is true, whatever is noble, whatever is right, whatever is pure, whatever is lovely, whatever is admirable—if anything is excellent or praiseworthy—think about such things."

It is a sin for a married person to think about having sexual relations with another; it is just as much a sin for an unmarried person to have fantasies about having sexual intercourse with another. In *The Act of Marriage* I list several steps for overcoming this temptation.

The first step is to confess all evil thinking as sin (1 John 1:9). Step two is to walk in the Spirit (Galatians 5:16—25). Step three is to ask God for victory (1 John 5:14—15). Step four is to avoid all suggestive materials that would provoke sinful thoughts. Step five: If married, think only about your spouse; if single, get your mind under control by thinking only pure thoughts about others. Step six: Repeat the first five for as long as it takes for your thoughts to come under submission.

FOREPLAY

Foreplay is the activity of kissing, hugging, and massaging as a man and woman prepare for intercourse. It is a time of closeness, warmth, and sharing in the most intimate expression of love between husband and wife.

Many people don't realize that men and women have different levels of arousal. A man can be sexually aroused and ready for intercourse within minutes, but a woman's desire is slowly intensified during foreplay until she is ready to give herself totally in sexual intercourse. Foreplay should be an unhurried time of relaxation, gentleness, and concern. Both husband and wife should be more concerned about making one's partner happy than about one's own desires. Only with this selfless attitude can the act of marriage truly be mutually satisfying.

FREQUENCY

There is no "correct" number of times that a husband and wife should have sexual intercourse each month or week. The frequency is a matter of personal preference mutually agreed upon by husband and wife. In the surveys I have seen, the average is from two to three times a week. That doesn't mean a husband and wife are "abnormal" if their lovemaking is more or less. I would question the health of a marriage, however, if a husband and wife seldom or never make love. The act of marriage is a good indicator of the love a man and woman have for each other. The desire to "become one" in sexual intercourse should be frequently present in a good marriage.

HOMOSEXUALITY / LESBIANISM

A heterosexual is a person who has a sexual preference for the opposite sex. Throughout man's cultural history and in the world of nature, this is God's approved order for the replenishing of the species on earth. It is the standard by which psychologists and psychiatrists *at one time* measured all other sexual conduct. The average heterosexual male and female were considered "normal," and any sexual conduct that deviated from this standard was considered "abnormal" or a "perversion." Until 1973 the *Diagnostic and Statistical Manual* of the American Psychiatric Association listed "homosexuality" as a sexual abnormality, a deviation that needed to be treated or cured.

But under pressure from an increasingly radicalized homosexual movement, the American Psychiatric Association removed homosexuality from its "abnormal" listing in 1973. In humanistic circles, homosexuality is now viewed as an alternate lifestyle, not as a sin or sexual perversion. Changing the definitions of words, however, does not change the reality.

There are no scientific studies of which I am aware that

demonstrate that homosexuals are born with a disposition to choose a member of their own sex. In doing research for my book *What Everyone Should Know About Homosexuality*, it became obvious to me that homosexuality is a *learned* behavior. There are certain factors that *predispose* some people toward homosexuality, but there is no genetic or hormonal cause for it.

Homosexuality in either men or women is essentially unnatural. God created males and females among human beings and animals with complementary sexual organs designed for the procreation of new life. Grace Ketterman observes that "since the biological purpose of sex is reproduction, homosexuality may be considered biologically abnormal to some degree, because its purpose is never reproduction. Homosexuality is extremely rare in the animal world."[3] Because we live in a fallen world, there are going to be exceptions to and corruptions of God's natural order among people and other living creatures. But these occasional sexual perversions should not be accepted as "alternate lifestyles."

In my book on homosexuality, I plotted the sequence whereby a person learns to become a homosexual. This is the progression: (1) A predisposition toward homosexuality; (2) an initial homosexual experience; (3) pleasurable and positive homosexual thoughts; (4) more homosexual experiences; (5) more pleasurable thoughts; (6) homosexuality.

Homosexual behavior is one of the most difficult perversions to cure. But there is hope. Homosexuals need, first of all, a changed inner nature that can come only from repentance for sins and acceptance of salvation in Jesus Christ. If you know of someone struggling with the problem of homosexuality, you might consult your church for the names and addresses of organizations that can help him.

IMPOTENCE

During the last twenty years more and more men have experienced difficulties in completing the act of marriage. If impotence is on the rise, it is undoubtedly not due to physical problems, but to thought patterns and stress factors that hinder a good sexual relationship. Most doctors whom I have talked with believe that impotence is caused by the intense emotional and career pressures of our present culture. Our world is far more insecure than it was twenty to thirty years ago. Men are less sure of themselves in their traditional role as head of the household. This self-doubt has led several writers to analyze the phenomenon of the "feminized male." With the women's liberation movement still generating sex-role confusion, we may expect even more sexual dysfunction among men in the years ahead.

MASTURBATION

The word *masturbation* comes from the Latin *masturbari,* which means to pollute oneself. Masturbation is variously described as "autoeroticism," "self-abuse," "self-pleasuring," or, in slang terms, "jacking off" or "jerking off." In males it refers to the practice of manipulating the penis until ejaculation occurs. In females, masturbation refers to the manipulation of the vulva and clitoris to achieve sexual stimulation.

Dr. Mary Calderone, former medical director of Planned Parenthood and founder of the humanistic Sex Information and Education Council of the United States (SIECUS), has co-authored a book entitled *Talking With Your Child About Sex.* This book states that children should be encouraged from the moment of birth to fondle their genitals and to masturbate or engage in "self-pleasuring." She and her co-author, James Ramey, comment that ". . . it has become clear to us that society must cease trying to interfere with the child's natural discovery and enjoyment of self-pleasuring."[4] I strongly disagree with Mary Calderone's humanistic viewpoint on sexual matters.

Masturbation is one of the most controversial sexual

subjects in the Christian community. The various opinions range from the viewpoint that masturbation is a marvelous gift of God to the view that it is a sin to be conquered by a Spirit-controlled believer. The Bible is silent on the subject, but we can draw certain principles from Scripture that might give us guidance.

1. We should keep in mind that masturbation is usually accompanied by lustful thoughts. In Matthew 5:28 Jesus tells us that a man can commit adultery in his heart by thinking lustfully about a woman.

2. Masturbation is often psychologically and physically addicting. Every pornography magazine on the market caters to the masturbatory inclinations of men. But when sexual desires are misdirected into a thought-life filled with lust and adultery, only spiritual harm can come to the man who finds himself in this bondage.

3. Sexual intercourse is designed by God to be enjoyed by a husband and wife in marriage. Often a man who is a chronic masturbator ends up preferring pornography and masturbation to sexual intercourse with his wife. It defrauds her of her rights as a sexual being.

4. Guilt invariably accompanies masturbatory fantasies. This guilt can inhibit spiritual growth.

MENOPAUSE

Menopause is also called the "change of life" in women and usually occurs over a five-year period of time from around ages forty-five to fifty. During this time a woman's menstrual cycle and monthly period become irregular and stop. A woman in her forties will begin to notice increasing irregularities in her cycle. This comes from a gradual decrease in the estrogen produced by her ovaries. Once menopause is complete, no more eggs are released for fertilization and a woman can bear no more children.

The irregularities in the cycle result from changes in the lining of the uterus. Some women experience fatigue, headaches, and mood swings called "hot flashes." There may be a noticeable sagging of the breasts, broadening of the hips, and an increasing weight problem. The emotional problems that may accompany menopause can be controlled by taking estrogen as prescribed by a physician. This allows a woman to go through menopause with a minimum of discomfort or extreme mood swings.

During menopause, many husbands and wives automatically assume that no more eggs are being produced so they have sexual intercourse without contraceptives. This often results in what doctors have called "change-of-life babies." Experts suggest that a woman wait at least two years into menopause before all contraceptives are discarded.

Men also experience a "menopause" of sorts, but it is usually not as difficult for them as for women. Usually in their late fifties men experience hormone changes that result in headaches, nervousness, fatigue, and other symptoms.

Both men and women often fear that they will lose their sexual potency as they go through the change of life. This frequently depends on their attitudes. There are no physical reasons why a man and woman should lose their sexual desires, but fear and anxiety often produce frigidity or impotence. A good mental attitude is the best medicine to cure any sexual difficulties after the change of life. Much research indicates that menopause even improves the sexual relations between a husband and wife because there are no anxieties about bearing children. The change of life in no way affects a woman's femininity or a man's masculine characteristics.

Sometimes sexual intercourse can be more painful for a woman after menopause because the vaginal walls have become thinner. But she can minimize the problem by taking sufficient estrogen or applying a vaginal cream. I point out in *The Act of Marriage*, "It has been conclusively shown that women who have satisfying sexual intercourse once or twice a week all through the menopausal years have fewer symptoms of hot flashes, irritability, nervousness, and much less change in the vaginal walls even with little or no hormone replacement."[5]

MENSTRUATION

Menstruus is a Latin word that means "monthly." Menstruation is the monthly discharge of a bloody fluid from a woman's uterus. It is the first visible sign that a girl is becoming sexually mature, capable of conceiving a child. The monthly menstrual cycle is also called a "period" and is usually completed in twenty-eight days.

The onset of the menstrual cycle, called **menarche,** is part of the body's maturation in changing a child into an adult over a four-or-five-year period of time known as adolescence. A girl's first period can begin anywhere between the ages nine and seventeen. Adolescence and the accompanying sex changes are all triggered by the master gland, the pituitary, that begins secreting hormones into other organs.

The menstrual cycle is a woman's monthly preparation for child bearing. The ovaries begin manufacturing estrogen, which is one of the primary hormones involved in maturing physically. Estrogen also causes a rapid development of the lining of the uterus in preparation for a fertilized egg. The lining fills with blood, waiting for the egg to implant itself in the wall. As soon as the egg attaches itself to the wall, the placenta develops and the blood begins supplying the needed nourishment to the human embryo. If the egg is not fertilized, the blood supply diminishes and millions of cells in the uterus wall die and are soon discarded in the menstrual flow. The fluid discarded from the uterus is actually half blood and half mucus and pieces of the uterine wall that are not needed.

The menstrual cycle lasts for thirty to thirty-five years until menopause.

NUDITY

While many humanistic psychologists and psychiatrists promote nudity in families, I believe the Scriptures and common sense make it obvious that parents should not allow themselves to be seen in the nude by their children. I agree with Dr. Melvin Anchell, who has written,

> Small children enjoy exposing their bodies or seeing others in the nude. This is a perfectly normal pleasure for the five year old. If the parents are neither prudish nor unduly immodest, children progress naturally from this early stage and learn normal modesty, by example.

> However, parents who lack a normal amount of modesty and persist in walking about nude, overly excite (and encourage) the child to see nudity and exhibit his own anatomy.

> A child may become permanently arrested in the exhibitionist-voyeur stage if he is seduced by an adult who derives sensual pleasure from exhibiting his anatomy to the child or viewing the child's anatomy. The sense of sight becomes eroticized, and erotic energies are abnormally released through this channel, the eye.[6]

Many parents mistakenly believe that they will create wholesome attitudes toward sex in their children if they openly display their sex organs. But what usually happens is that the child becomes morbidly obsessed with sexual matters and may develop voyeuristic tendencies or begin fantasizing about having sexual relations with his or her parent. This may also lead to sexual experimentation with playmates. One psychoanalyst observed that parents who walk about in the nude in front of their children are unconsciously seducing their own children.

Many passages of Scripture deal with nakedness or nudity. Before the Fall in the Garden of Eden, Adam and Eve were naked and felt no shame. No sin was connected with their nudity; they were pure in the sight of God. But when they sinned, they immediately clothed themselves because they felt ashamed and fearful. Since the Fall, the Bible condemns physical nakedness, especially among family members. In Genesis 9 we are told that Noah planted a vineyard, got drunk, and lay in his tent naked. One of his sons, Ham, discovered his nakedness and told Japheth and Shem about it. Shem and Japheth put a garment on their shoulders, *backed* into the tent so as to avoid seeing their father in such a condition, and covered him. They turned their faces away in respect to their father.

In Leviticus, God expressly forbids the Jews from exposing the nakedness of their relatives. Chapter 18 is devoted to this subject. Verse 10 states, "You must not have sexual relations with your son's daughter or your daughter's daughter; their nakedness you shall not uncover, for they are your own flesh" (AMPLIFIED).

Nakedness also has a spiritual meaning in Scripture. It refers to sin being exposed or shameful acts being revealed. In Isaiah 47:3 the Lord says, "Your nakedness shall be exposed, and your shame shall be seen. I will take vengeance, and I will spare no man—none I encounter (will be able to resist Me)" (AMPLIFIED).

The New Testament tells of the demoniac of Gadara who lived naked among the caves, cutting himself with rocks. When Jesus healed him, he sat at Jesus's feet, "dressed and in his right mind" (Mark 5:15).

In our culture, public nudity provokes lustful thoughts and leads people into sin. In other cultures, where lust has not been marketed like a product, nudity is not a major issue—but Christian morality is not an issue either.

Wise parents should teach their children to be modest in their dress and behavior. Nudity outside the bedroom should have no place in a Christian home. I realize that occasionally a parent will be caught off guard and be seen in the nude, but when that happens, the reaction should be calmness and discretion with a move to covering as soon as possible.

ORAL SEX

In counseling Christians I hear as many questions about oral sex as on any other subject. Like masturbation, this subject is controversial in the Christian community. What is oral sex? One term, **fellatio,** refers to the act of a woman receiving the penis in her mouth to sexually stimulate the male. In **cunnilingus,** the male stimulates the woman with his mouth over her vulva area, often with his tongue on her clitoris. Both acts can bring orgasm if prolonged.

I do not recommend the practice of oral sex, but admittedly there are no biblical grounds for forbidding it. It appears to be a matter of personal preference. There is one major consequence if it is practiced promiscuously. Herpes Simplex II is a venereal disease caused by a cold-sore virus that has become a national epidemic during recent years. One college counselor has observed that this disease is widely spread through oral-genital sexual encounters. Oral sex has been popularized in the last ten years through a variety of men's and women's magazines, and it seems to be the sexual "fad" of the 1980s. More than 20 million Americans now have this incurable "genital herpes."

Some Christians justify oral sex on the basis of Hebrews 13:4, which states, "Marriage should be honored by all, and the marriage bed kept pure, for God will judge the adulterer and all the sexually immoral." They say that "anything married couples do in bed is all right." This kind of reasoning does injustice to the original language. The Greek word for "bed" is *coitay,* from which we get the English word "coitus," meaning intercourse. Literally this verse says, "Marriage is honorable in all and coitus is undefiled." Obviously that does not give a scriptural endorsement of oral sex. I do not recommend oral sex for Christians.

ORGASMIC FAILURE

Dr. David Reuben, author of *Everything You Always Wanted to Know About Sex,* uses the term "orgasmic impairment" to describe a woman's inability to achieve an orgasm during lovemaking.[7] The woman's clitoris, as explained earlier, is the sexual trigger and the equivalent of a penis. If this organ is tenderly manipulated by the husband with his finger or with his penis, his wife will usually experience orgasm.

Unfortunately, some men and women still suffer from lack of information regarding the mechanics of sexual love. I believe misconception and misinformation about orgasm are the main causes of sexual malfunction among women. It was once thought that a woman should not have an orgasm— that it was only the privilege of a husband to experience sexual release. Fortunately our ideas have changed, but guilt feelings remain for some women. These feelings can significantly impair a woman's enjoyment of sex.

Fear is another cause of orgasmic failure. Sometimes a woman is afraid she won't perform as well as she should, and as a result she doesn't.

In counseling engaged or married couples I try to allay whatever guilt or fear they may have regarding sexual intercourse. I tell them that the act of marriage is God-ordained and God-blessed and the highest physical expression of love between a husband and wife. The marriage bed is to be a place of joy, free from inhibitions—the one place where modesty is to be shunned if a man and woman are to experience the full blessings of sexual love.

PETTING

The term *petting* refers to kissing, hugging, and body rubbing that take place between a boy and girl on a date. Petting is actually foreplay, or the activity that prepares a couple for sexual intercourse. During petting, a boy will usually massage a girl's breasts and genitals; a girl will rub his sex organs. This is risky, because it leads both the girl and boy toward sexual intercourse. If petting is stopped just before intercourse, frustration and guilt may result. Pregnancy, venereal diseases, guilt, fear, and loss of respect or self-respect are all potential consequences of unrestrained petting.

PORNOGRAPHY

The word *pornography* refers to material that is sexually explicit, erotic, and offensive—whether it be movies, magazines, TV programs, books, videotapes, or other forms of communication. "Pornography" comes from two Greek words, *porneia,* which is translated "fornication" or "immorality" in the Bible, and *graphos,* which refers to writing. Together these two words literally mean "writing about harlots."

It is important to differentiate between pornography and legal obscenity. Something that is pornographic may not necessarily be *legally* obscene as defined by the U.S. Supreme Court in *Miller v. California* in 1973. For obscene material to be prosecuted and banned, a jury must judge whether the pornographic material under consideration fulfills the *Miller* definition of "obscenity." Magazines such as *Playboy, Penthouse,* and *Hustler* are pornographic because they focus on the activities of women who are selling their bodies or prostituting themselves for money.

Pornography is one of the most serious social scourges of our nation and is currently an $8-billion-a-year industry. We have seen rising levels of venereal disease, child sexual abuse, homosexuality, divorce, rape, and social deterioration in America because of the spread of pornography. Only tough, consistent law enforcement, citizen action, and prayer will rid our country of this psychological venereal disease.

PROSTITUTION

Prostitutes are people who provide sexual services for money or other material gain.

RAPE

Rape is a violent sexual act usually perpetrated against women by men. In rape, a man forces a woman to have sexual intercourse with him. In many cases he also brutalizes or kills her. The man who rapes is usually an angry person who has a poor self-image. He rapes in order to feel a sense of power or revenge against those he believes have hurt him in the past. It is not so much an act of self-gratification as a psychological weapon. It is probably the most physically and emotionally traumatic experience a woman can ever endure.

Women who have been raped need spiritual counsel to overcome their feelings of guilt and uncleanness. Often rape victims blame themselves for being raped instead of placing the blame where it rightfully belongs—on the cruel rapist and the greedy pornographer whose products may stimulate the rapist toward his crime.

SEX DRIVE

The God-given sex drive in men and women is a blessing as long as it is kept under control. We are sexual creatures with an innate desire to procreate. This desire is properly fulfilled only within the bonds of marriage.

For the unmarried, the sex drive must be "sublimated," or rechanneled into constructive pursuits. Sublimated sexual energy has contributed to the great progress and resourcefulness of the United States in technology and industry. It formed the basis of what has come to be known as "the Protestant work ethic." Pleasure-seeking or sexual dissipation was frowned upon, but hard work was highly approved. Social scientists who have studied fallen civilizations note that these cultures declined as strict controls on sexual energy were relaxed. Nations with permissive sexual standards invariably declined.

Sexual drive within marriage is a variable thing, depending on people's temperament, background, and general energy level. Some mates seem to lack any sex drive; others are seemingly never satisfied. The frequency of sexual relations between a husband and wife should be mutually agreed upon.

SEX SLANG

Some people have a habit of using vulgar words to describe what God has given to us as a beautiful union between husband and wife. Sexual slang words are used as curses or statements of violence against others. It would not be appropriate to mention specific vulgar sexual terms in this book. I do not believe any Spirit-led Christian should use these terms.

SEXUAL INTERCOURSE

Sexual intercourse is the act of marriage. During this union, a man places his penis inside a woman's vagina. Using his pelvic muscles, he thrusts in and out until sperm ejaculates from the penis into the vagina. Sexual intercourse is God's design for the reproduction of the species. It is also a way for a husband and wife to express their love toward each other; it is designed for their enjoyment.

TRANSVESTISM / TRANSEXUALITY

A transvestite is a person—usually a man—who dresses and behaves like the opposite sex. Because he feels he should have been born the other gender, he is uncomfortable with his sexuality so he begins to wear women's clothing and assume feminine mannerisms. These people are not homosexuals, and many of them are married with children; but they secretly wish to be women.

Some transvestites decide to have sex-change operations to make them into females. Thus they become "trans-sexuals." Through hormonal therapy and operations, they eventually look like females, but they are unable to bear children.

WET DREAMS

A "wet dream," more formally called a "nocturnal emission," refers to the ejaculation of sperm from the penis while a male is asleep. Every day the testicles manufacture sperm that accumulate in tubes and small storage areas in the body. When these storage spaces are filled, the male experiences a need for sexual release. In a uniquely designed system, God has made an "escape valve" for the sperm through wet dreams. The male who experiences a nocturnal emission usually has a sexually oriented dream, but this should be no cause for guilt feelings; no one can control the content of his dreams. Wet dreams are usually disturbing to boys in puberty unless their parents have prepared them properly so they know in advance what to expect.

Glossary

ADOLESCENCE—The time in a person's life that generally parallels the teenage years. Beginning with puberty, when the sexual organs mature, this is a time of transition from childhood to adulthood.

ADULTERY—Sexual intercourse between two people who are not married to each other.

AMNIOTIC FLUID—The watery fluid that surrounds and protects the fetus as it grows in the mother's womb.

AMNIOTIC SAC—The tough but elastic bag that holds the growing fetus and the amniotic fluid. When the baby is ready to be born, this sac breaks open and the amniotic fluid flows out of the uterus and vagina. When this happens, the mother's "water has broken."

AMPULLA CHAMBER—The storage chamber for sperm that have left the epididymis and traveled through the vas deferens.

ANDROGEN—The hormone that produces sexual changes in a boy, including the growth of the sex drive, body hair, and a deepened voice.

CERVIX—The small opening at the bottom of the uterus that connects with the birth canal, or vagina. This opening is usually only the size of pencil lead but expands many times when the baby is ready to be born.

CHASTITY—Abstinence from premarital or extramarital sexual intercourse. Purity in conduct and intention.

CHROMOSOMES—Tiny threadlike bodies in each cell that contain the genetic blueprints for each person. Sperm cells contain twenty-three chromosomes, and ova twenty-three. When an egg is fertilized by a sperm cell, the combined forty-six chromosomes determine the hair color, temperament, facial features, body build, and hundreds of other characteristics of the developing child.

CIRCUMCISION—A surgical procedure, usually performed for hygienic or religious reasons within a few days after a boy is born, in which the loose skin (the foreskin) covering the end of the penis is removed.

CLIMAX—See *Orgasm*.

CONCEPTION—The moment in which a new life is created when a sperm cell burrows its way into and fertilizes an egg.

CONTRACEPTION—Various methods that have been devised to prevent the conception of new life. The birth-control pill is a contraceptive device that prevents ovulation. The condom, or "safe," is a contraceptive that prevents sperm from entering the vagina.

COWPER'S GLAND—The first sexual gland to function when a man is sexually aroused. It sends a slippery fluid through the urethra to neutralize the acids of the urine. Once the acid is neutralized, the sperm can pass through the urethra unharmed.

EJACULATION—The forceful expulsion of sperm and semen from the penis. The male orgasm.

EMBRYO—The unborn baby during the first eight weeks of development. After the eighth week, the baby is called a fetus.

ENDOMETRIUM—The soft, furlike lining that develops on the wall of the uterus. During a woman's menstrual period, this lining fills with blood in preparation to receive a fertilized egg. When no egg is fertilized, the lining dissolves and is discharged through the vagina. If a fertilized egg embeds itself in the lining, the endometrium becomes part of the placenta.

ENDOCRINE SYSTEM—Glands in the male and female bodies that secrete powerful hormones into the bloodstream, controlling the activity of organs or tissues in another part of the body.

EPIDIDYMIS—A mass of small coiled tubes just above the testicles. Inside, the sperm cells mature before passing through the spermatic duct (vas deferens) into the ampulla chamber and seminal vesicles.

ERECTION—The state of sexual arousal in which the penis fills with blood and becomes stiff and ready for intercourse and ejaculation.

ESTROGEN—A powerful female hormone that is secreted by the ovary and placenta during puberty, the menstrual cycle, and pregnancy. It stimulates secondary female characteristics such as breast development.

FALLOPIAN TUBE—The two tubes (also called oviducts) that lead from the ovaries into the uterus, or womb. Each month an egg, released from one of the ovaries, makes its way through the Fallopian tube, where fertilization can take place. The egg proceeds to the uterus either fertilized or unfertilized.

FERTILIZATION—Conception.

FETUS—A developing life in the womb after the eighth week. The word means "young one."

FORESKIN—Loose skin that covers the head of the penis (glans penis). This foreskin is normally removed by circumcision shortly after a boy's birth.

FORNICATION—Sexual intercourse between unmarried men and women.

GENE—A unit in a chromosome that carries a particular physical characteristic.

GENITALS—The reproductive or sexual organs of a man or woman.

GLANS PENIS—The head of the penis, comprising densely packed nerves, which is one of the most sensitive areas of a man's body and when stimulated will promote ejaculation.

HEREDITY—The transmission of physical and emotional traits to children through the combination of a man and woman's chromosomes.

HETEROSEXUAL—A man or woman who is attracted to members of the opposite sex. Heterosexuality is evidence of normal sexuality in men and women.

HOMOSEXUAL—A sexual deviation in which a person is attracted to members of his or her own sex. God's Word refers to homosexual behavior as sin; modern psychologists and humanistic teachers refer to homosexuality as an "alternate lifestyle."

HORMONE—A chemical produced by an endocrine gland that affects other organs or tissues within the body. Certain hormones promote male or female characteristics.

HYMEN—A membrane on the back part of the outside opening of the vagina. The opening of the hymen (also called the maidenhead) in a virgin is about one inch in diameter.

INTERCOURSE—The "act of marriage" between a man and a woman. Intercourse occurs when a man places his penis inside the woman's vagina in lovemaking. Sexual intercourse is only to take place in the bonds of marriage. Sexual activity outside of marriage is fornication or adultery.

LESBIAN—A female homosexual.

LIBIDO—The desire for sexual activity present in males and females, also known as the sex drive.

MASTURBATION—Self-stimulation of the sexual organs. A man rubs his penis until he ejaculates; the woman manipulates her clitoris until she has an orgasm.

MENSTRUATION—The passage of the endometrium and blood from the uterus through the vagina during a woman's monthly period. The menstrual period occurs every twenty-eight days.

NAVEL—The shriveled remains of the umbilical cord on a baby after the cord has been severed from the mother.

NOCTURNAL EMISSION—The unconscious act (also called a "wet dream") by which a male's body disposes of excess sperm. The emission normally occurs during sleep as the penis becomes erect and expels sperm that are too numerous to store in the various tubes and sacs of a male's genital system. The emission is often accompanied by a sexual dream.

ORGASM—The climax of sexual intercourse. In males it occurs when sperm are forcefully ejaculated from the penis; in females it occurs when the clitoris is properly stimulated to produce a highly intense sexual sensation.

OVARY—Either of two female organs near the kidneys that produce ova (egg cells) and the hormone estrogen, which governs feminine characteristics. Each month a mature egg cell is released from one ovary and passing through a Fallopian tube to await fertilization.

OVULATION—The process of discharging an egg cell from the ovary.

OVUM—An egg cell.

PENIS—The spongy, tubelike male sex organ that serves a dual purpose in at times eliminating waste water and at times ejaculating sperm.

PERIOD—The three-to-five days during the month when a woman is experiencing menstruation (the shedding of the endometrium).

PITUITARY—The master gland at the base of the brain that secretes hormones affecting growth, sexual development, and the functioning of other glands: the adrenals, sex glands, and thyroid.

PLACENTA—A spongy organ attached to the wall of the uterus and connected to a fetus by an umbilical cord. Filled with blood veins, this organ filters food and oxygen through the umbilical cord and disposes of waste products from the fetus. Also called the afterbirth.

PREGNANCY—The period of time between conception and the birth of the child, approximately 266 days in length, or roughly nine months. From a Latin word meaning "previous to bringing forth."

PROGESTERONE—A chemical, often referred to as the "pregnancy hormone," that is secreted by the ovaries and prepares the lining of the uterus for the placenta and fetus. It also prevents further menstruation and ovulation during pregnancy.

PROSTATE—A gland located near the urethra and bladder that secretes part of a male's seminal fluid. It is not uncommon in old age for the prostate to enlarge, impede urination, and require surgical removal.

PUBERTY—The period of time in a child's life (beginning anytime between age nine and seventeen) when he or she begins to mature sexually.

REPRODUCTION—The process of producing offspring that are basically the same as the parents.

SCROTUM—The sac of skin that hangs behind the man's penis and contains the testicles, which produce male hormones and sperm cells.

SEMEN—A fluid that contains the sperm cells. Semen is ejaculated from the penis when the male is engaged in sexual intercourse. It comprises secretions from the testicles, prostate, seminal vesicles, and Cowper's glands.

SEMINAL EMISSIONS—See *Nocturnal emissions.*

SEMINAL VESICLES—Two storage areas for sperm, located on either side of the prostate, that are connected to the sperm duct, or vas deferens.

SEXUAL INTERCOURSE— See *Intercourse.*

SEXUAL ORGANS—The male or female reproductive organs.

SPERM—The mature male reproductive cell that fertilizes the female ovum.

SYPHILIS—See *Venereal disease.*

TESTICLES—Two almond-shaped organs inside the scrotum that manufacture millions of sperm cells and produce testosterone, the male hormone responsible for secondary sex characteristics in males (such as voice change and body hair).

TESTOSTERONE—A male sex hormone produced in the testicles that produces secondary sex characteristics in males during puberty.

TRICHOMONIASIS—See *Venereal disease.*

UMBILICAL CORD—The cord that connects the fetus to the placenta in the mother's uterus. Through the cord, which comprises two arteries and a vein, the baby receives nourishment and oxygen and expels waste material through the mother's system.

URETHRA—In both males and females, the tube used to eliminate urine or waste water from the body. In the male, it is also the passageway through which sperm cells are ejaculated during intercourse.

UTERUS—The pear-shaped organ in the mother's body that holds the developing embryo and fetus. It is one of the largest muscles in the body.

VAGINA—A woman's birth canal. The passageway from the cervix (bottom portion of the uterus) to the vulva (the external sex organs). During intercourse, the man's penis is placed inside the vagina.

VENEREAL DISEASE—Any of a variety of contagious diseases normally transmitted by intimate sexual contact, especially promiscuous activity. Commonly referred to now as "Sexually transmitted disease," VD can include gonorrhea, herpes simplex II, nongonococcal urethritis (NGU), syphilis, trichomoniasis, monilia, venereal warts, crabs, scabies, and AIDS (Acquired Immune Deficiency Syndrome). Some are medically treatable and some are not.

VIRGIN—A male or female who has never experienced sexual intercourse.

VULVA—The external female sexual organs, including the clitoris, labia majora, and labia minora.

WET DREAM—See *Nocturnal emission.*

WOMB—See *Uterus.*

X CHROMOSOME—A sex-determining chromosome found in both males and females. A female's eggs contain only X chromosones; half of a male's sperm contain X chromosomes and the other half have Y. When an X-chromosome sperm fertilizes an egg, the child becomes a female.

Y CHROMOSOME—A sex-determining chromosome found only in the male sperm. If a Y chromosome sperm fertilizes an X-chromosome egg, the child becomes a male.

Notes

CHAPTER 2

[1]Carol Atwater, "It Can Get Pretty Lively in the Womb," *U.S.A. Today* (August 2, 1983): 1–2D.
[2]Ibid.
[3]Ibid.
[4]George E. Gardner, *The Emerging Personality: Infancy Through Adolescence* (New York: Delacorte Press, 1970), 24.
[5]George A. Rekers, *Growing Up Straight* (Chicago: Moody Press, 1982), 38–39.
[6]Gardner, *The Emerging Personality*, 52.
[7]Grace H. Ketterman, *How to Teach Your Child About Sex* (Old Tappan, N.J.: Fleming H. Revell, 1981), 8.

CHAPTER 3

[1]Selma H. Fraiberg, *The Magic Years: Understanding and Handling the Problems of Early Childhood* (New York: Scribners, 1984), 59.
[2]Gardner, *The Emerging Personality*, 92.
[3]Raymond Moore and Dorothy S. Moore, *Better Late Than Early: A New Approach to Your Child's Education* (Berrien Springs, Mich.: Reader's Digest Press, 1982).
[4]Clyde M. Narramore, *Understanding Your Children*, (Grand Rapids: Zondervan, 1978), 123.
[5]W. Peter Blitchington, *Sex Roles and the Christian Family* (Wheaton, Ill.: Tyndale House Publishers, 1984), 107.

CHAPTER 4

[1]Frances Ilg and Louis Ames, *Child Behavior* (New York: Perennial Library, 1955), 3.
[2]Gary Bergel, *When You Were Formed in Secret* (Elyria, Ohio: Intercessors for Life, 1980), 1–13.

CHAPTER 5

[1]Tim LaHaye and Beverly LaHaye, *The Act of Marriage* (Grand Rapids: Zondervan, 1976), 269–70.
[2]James C. Dobson, *Preparing for Adolescence* (Ventura, Calif.: Vision House, 1978), 86–87.
[3]Blitchington, *Sex Roles and the Christian Family*, 51.
[4]Tim LaHaye, *The Battle for the Family* (Old Tappan, N.J.: Fleming H. Revell, 1982), 17.
[5]Carl Wilson, *Our Dance Has Turned to Death* (Wheaton, Ill.: Tyndale House, 1979), 84–85.
[6]Tim LaHaye, *What Everyone Should Know About Homosexuality* (Wheaton, Ill.: Tyndale House, 1980).
[7]Ibid., 78.
[8]Rekers, *Growing Up Straight*, 75.

CHAPTER 7

[1]Nadine Broznan, "Witness Says She Fears 'Child Predator' Network," *New York Times* (18 September 1984): A21.
[2]Clifford Linedecker, *Children in Chains* (New York: Everest House, 1981), 119.
[3]Interim Report, Sixty-sixth Legislative Session, Select Committee on Pornography: Its Related Causes and Control (Washington), 21–22.
[4]Linedecker, *Children in Chains*, 32.
[5]Shirley O'Brien, *Child Pornography* (Dubusque, Ia.: Kendall/Hunt Publishing Co., 1983), 9.
[6]Ibid., 83.
[7]Joan Sweeney, "The Child Molester: No Profile," *Los Angeles Times* (25 April 1984), 1.
[8]O'Brien, *Child Pornography,* 139.

CHAPTER 9

[1]Carl Wilson, *Our Dance Has Turned to Death,* 132.
[2]Gerhard Hauer, *Longing for Tenderness* (Downers Grove, Ill.: InterVarsity Press, 1983), 2.
[3]Herbert Miles, *Sexual Understanding Before Marriage* (Grand Rapids: Zondervan, 1971), 66.
[4]Blitchington, *Sex Roles and the Christian Family,* 152.
[5]Virginia Watts Smith, *The Single Parent,* rev. ed. (Old Tappan, N.J.: Fleming H. Revell, Power Books, 1983).

CHAPTER 11

[1]Eric W. Johnson, *V.D.* (Philadelphia: J. B. Lippincott, 1978), 7.
[2]Ibid., 71.
[3]*USA Today* (December 13, 1984): 6A.
[4]"S.F. Health Chief Resigns, Blames Anti-AIDS Drive," *San Diego Union* (December 12, 1984): A3.
[5]*USA Today* (December 13, 1984): 6A.
[6]*Time* (July 4, 1983).
[7]William Marberry and Hollis Wood, "Activist Attorney Robert Schwab Is AIDS Victim," *Dallas–Fort Worth Gay News* (May 20, 1983).

CHAPTER 12

[1]Ketterman, *How to Teach Your Child About Sex,* 153.
[2]LaHaye and LaHaye, *The Act of Marriage,* 189–90.
[3]Ketterman, *How to Teach Your Children About Sex,* 167.
[4]Mary Calderone and James Ramey, *Talking With Your Child About Sex* (New York: Ballantine, 1982), xv.
[5]LaHaye and LaHaye, *The Act of Marriage,* 273.
[6]Melvin Anchell, *Sex and Insanity* (Portland, Ore.: Halcyon House, 1983), 79–80.
[7]David Reuben, *Everything You Always Wanted to Know About Sex But Were Afraid to Ask* (New York: Bantam, 1971).